Child Health in the Tropics

A practical handbook for health personnel

Edited by D.B. Jelliffe

MD, FRCP, FAAP, FAPHA, DCH, DTM & H
Professor of Paediatrics and Public Health, University of
California, Los Angeles, California, USA; formerly Director,
Caribbean Food and Nutrition Institute, Kingston, Jamaica;
formerly Professor of Paediatrics and Child Health, Makerere
Medical School, Kampala, Uganda; Visiting Professor of Tropical
Medicine, Tulane University, New Orleans, USA

Fifth edition

Edward Arnold

© D.B. Jelliffe 1985

First published 1962
by Edward Arnold (Publishers) Ltd
41 Bedford Square, London WC1B 3DQ

Edward Arnold (Australia) Pty Ltd, 80 Waverley Road,
Caulfield East, Victoria 3145, Australia

Edward Arnold, 300 North Charles Street, Baltimore,
Maryland 21201, U.S.A.

Reprinted 1963
Second edition 1964
Reprinted with amendments 1966
Third edition 1968
Reprinted 1969, 1970, 1972, (twice)
Fourth edition 1974
Reprinted 1975, 1978, 1979
Fifth edition 1985
Reprinted 1986

Spanish edition 1966
(Published by Pan American Health Organization, Washington DC)
Second Spanish edition 1974

ELBS edition first published 1975
Reprinted 1978, 1979

Child health in the Tropics.—5th ed,
1. Pediatric tropical medicine
I. Jelliffe, D.B.
613'.0432'0913   RJ47

ISBN 0-7131-4438-6

Text set in 10/11pt Times Compugraphic
by CK Typesetters Ltd, Sutton, Surrey.
Printed and bound in Great Britain by Richard Clay
(The Chaucer Press) Ltd, Bungay, Suffolk

Contributors

Ashfaq Ahmad FRCP, FCPS, FAAP, DCH
Professor and Head, Department of Paediatrics, Khyber Medical College, Peshawar, Pakistan

F. John Bennett MB, ChB, DPH, FFCM
Regional Advisor in Community Health, UNICEF, Nairobi, Kenya

John Biddulph MD
Professor of Paediatrics, University of Papua New Guinea, Port Moresby, Papua New Guinea

Nimrod Bwibo MB, ChB, FAAP, MPH, MRCP
Professor of Paediatrics, and Principal, College of Health Sciences, University of Nairobi, Kenya

Robert Cook MD
Senior Medical Officer, Family Health, World Health Organization, Geneva, Switzerland

Mamdouh M. Gabr MD, FRCP
Professor of Paediatrics, Head, Paediatric Department, Faculty of Medicine, Cairo University and Former Minister of Health, Cairo, Egypt.

Shanti Ghosh MB, BS, DCH, DTM & H
Formerly Head, Department of Paediatrics, Safdarjang Hospital, New Delhi, India

Michael Gurney
Senior Programme Officer, Nutrition Unit, World Health Organization, Geneva, Switzerland

Erasmus Harland MD
Formerly Professor of Paediatrics, University of the West Indies, Kingston, Jamaica; Head, Paediatric Department, Riyadh Armed Forces Hospital, Riyadh, Saudi Arabia

Contributors

Mahmoud Mohamed Hassan MD, FRCP, FAAP, DCH
Head, Paediatric Department, Maternity and Children's Hospital, Jeddah, Saudi Arabia

Sa'ad Hijazi MD, FAAP, DCH, PhD
Professor of Nutrition and Child Health; Dean, Faculty of Medicine, Yarmouk University, Irbid, Jordan

Aaron Ifekwunigwe MD, MRCP, DCH, MPH
Associate Professor, Department of Family Medicine, Charles Drew Graduate Medical School, Los Angeles, California, USA

Derrick B. Jelliffe MD, FCRP, FAAP, FAPHA, DCH, DTM & H
Professor of Paediatrics and Public Health, Division of Population and Family Health, School of Public Health, University of California, Los Angeles, California, USA

E.F. Patrice Jelliffe MPH, FRSH
Lecturer/Researcher, Division of Population and Family Health, School of Public Health, University of California, Los Angeles, California, USA

Charlotte G. Neumann MD, MPH
Professor, Department of Public Health and Paediatrics, School of Public Health and Medicine, University of California, Los Angeles, California, USA.

Susan Pettiss PhD
Formerly Director, Blindness Prevention, Helen Keller International, New York, N.Y., USA

Olikoye Ransome-Kuti MB, FRCP, FMC Paed.
Professor of Paediatrics, College of Medicine, University of Lagos, Lagos, Nigeria

Kusum Shah MD, DGO
Formerly Associate Professor of Obstetrics and Gynaecology, Grant Medical College and JJ Group of Government Hospitals, Bombay, India

P.M. Shah MD, DCH, FIAP, FICP
Medical Officer, Maternal and Child Health, World Health Organization, Geneva, Switzerland

Contributors

Hafiz el Shizali MB, BS, MD, FRCP, DCH
Professor, Department of Paediatrics, Medical School, University of Wad Medani, Wad Medani, Sudan

J. Paget Stanfield MD, FRCP, DCH
African Medical and Research Foundation, Nairobi, Kenya, East Africa

John Vince MB, ChB, FRCP, MD
Specialist Medical Officer, Paediatrics, Port Moresby General Hospital; Honorary Lecturer in Child Health, University of Papua New Guinea, Port Moresby, Papua New Guinea

Preface

In tropical countries, most of the population are children, among whom much unnecessary misery, disease and death occurs.

In plans which developing countries have for a healthier, more prosperous future, an obvious priority need for attention to be given to children — the next generation — continues as much as ever.

Much of the problem rests with improving social and economic conditions, particularly in striving to assure a fairer distribution of 'resources', including income, land and health services.

With the health service itself, considerable responsibility for the improvement of child care can rest with physicians or senior nurses, often working in difficult, remote rural areas with limited equipment, poor surroundings and sometimes with too little training or experience in tropical paediatrics, especially in community aspects of the subject.

At the same time, it is certain that, for the foreseeable future, the vast majority of child health work in rural areas and slums will, in fact, be carried out by various auxiliaries and village-level workers making up the 'primary health care services' (p.244, 247).

Hospitals need to play an important, but changing, role, with more emphasis on their use in health education (p.190), in carefully testing methods of treatment for use in rural areas, and for some special tests and forms of treatment.

However, all recent studies have shown that curative services alone are not going to improve matters. For this reason, increased emphasis has been given in the present edition to preventive services, including health education (p.190) and community participation (p.244), to the close link between the health of the mother and her offspring (p.6, 22),

Preface

to the training of primary health care workers (p.215), and to a brief mention of child health policy (p.251) — that is, how the governments plan to tackle health problems in children, mainly through ministries of health.

This edition has been thoroughly revised to include newer ideas on immunization (p.190) and oral rehydration (p.102), and to take into account such developments as the lack of response of some malarial parasites to some antimalarials, e.g. chloroquine (p.119), and the use of newer oral drugs to treat schistosomiasis (p.117). It now has authorship selected from leading experts from many regions of the world to increase its international perspective. Necessarily, however, this reflects occasional differences of opinion or experience.

The book is intended to cover the main aspects of child health — clinical, preventive and social — as seen all over the tropics, and to a lesser extent in poor, 'disadvantaged' areas in any part of the world, including industrialized countries.

Conditions of mainly clinical, hospital significance, such as diseases of the heart or kidneys, and conditions of local importance have not been covered. Examples of the latter include vitamin D deficiency, Chagas' disease, bladder stones, kala-azar, cancrum oris, yellow fever, dengue and cholera. Selection has been necessary to include problems with the widest distribution and consequences. These include, for example, diarrhoea (p.102), the main forms of malnutrition, including xerophthalmia (vitamin A deficiency, p.96), protein–energy malnutrition (PEM, p.65) and iron deficiency (p.83), combined with bacterial, viral and parasitic infections. Details cannot be covered in a small book, and the suggested reading list (p.275) gives reference to books in which further information can, and should, be sought, both on conditions covered and especially on problems that could not be included because of space limitations.

It is hoped that this brief account has been prepared in a suitable form for use selectively by medical and paramedical personnel — and especially by instructors and trainers of various types of staff working in primary health care services. It is, of course, not complete, but is intended as an introduction for physicians, senior nursing cadres and medical students, needing to be supplemented by much further reading (p.275). Also, considerable modification, simplification of language and adaption to the local situation will be needed for use in training primary health care workers (p.255).

Special thanks are due to Dr J. Paget Stanfield for advice on drug dosage.

1985   Derrick B. Jelliffe

Contents

Contents

Conversion tables

Imperial to metric
1 inch = 2.5 centimetres
1 foot = 30.5 centimetres
1 grain = 65 milligrams
1 ounce (avoirdupois) = 28.5 grams
1 pound (avoirdupois) = 454 grams = 0.454 kilograms
1 drachm = 3.5 millilitres
1 fluid ounce = 28 millilitres
1 pint (imperial — 20 fluid ounces) = 568 millilitres = 0.57 litres
1 gallon (imperial) = 4.55 litres

Metric to imperial
1 centimetre = 0.39 inches
1 metre = 3 feet 3¼ inches
100 milligrams = 1½ grains
1 gram = 15 grains
100 gram = 3½ ounces
1 kilogram = 35 ounces = 2.2 pounds
100 ml = 3½ ounces
1 litre = 35 fluid ounces = 1¾ pints (imperial)

1
Background

Derrick B. Jelliffe and E.F. Patrice Jelliffe

Tropical countries usually have 'young' populations, about half of which are children, among whom there is much ill-health.

  1. *Newborn* (first 28 days of life). The incidences of deaths and disease in newborn babies in the tropics are difficult to estimate. Both are certainly frequent, due to general infection (septicaemia) or tetanus of the newborn (p.37), to birth injury from unskilled midwifery (p.13), to lower birth weight (p.42), and to congenital abnormalities.

  2. *Infants* (first year of life). The infant mortality rate (or deaths in the first year of life per 1000 babies born alive) is high. In Europe and North America it is below 40. In tropical regions, it is often between 75 and 500 — that is, at least twice as high. However, it is difficult to measure accurately when births and deaths are not recorded, as is often the case in many countries, especially in rural areas.

  In the tropics, causes of death in infancy include those in the newborn (see above) and vary with the local situation (whether breast-fed or not, presence of malaria in the community etc.). Respiratory tract infection (especially pneumonia, p.124) is usually common. Diarrhoea (p.102) and nutritional marasmus (p.69) are often important, mainly in infants who are not breast-fed.

  3. *Preschool-age child* (1–4 years). Chief diseases in this age group in the tropics are protein–energy malnutrition (especially kwashiorkor, p.66), diarrhoea (p.102), pneumonia (p.132), malaria (p.117), those due to intestinal worms, (especially the hookworm and the roundworm, p.110), and whooping cough (p.165). Children in this age group are also at risk from accidents (p.187). Very frequently, preschool-age children suffer from several of these conditions at once.

There is a high death rate in this age group, often at least 20 times as great as in Europe and North America, largely from the combined effects of diseases which are preventable.

4. *Schoolchildren* (5–15 years). Although schoolchildren do not have the high mortality rate found in younger groups, they do have special problems, as well as opportunities (p.236). The main conditions often include moderate malnutrition, infectious diseases (such as tuberculosis, p.135), infestation with intestinal worms (p.110), attacks of malaria (p.117) and skin diseases (p.185).

Causes of childhood illness

The types of illness seen in children in different parts of the world depend to a considerable extent on the following.

Poverty, Hygiene and Education

If hygiene is poor (as judged by housing, water supply, and the disposal of excreta and rubbish), then illness will be common in all age groups, especially among children. For example, overcrowded houses help the spread of tuberculosis (p.135) and respiratory infections (p.124). A poor water supply results in children being dirty and developing various skin diseases (p.185) and diarrhoea (p.102). An absence of latrines, or a failure to use them, means that the ground will be soiled with stools, leading to the easy spread of intestinal worms (p.110). Poor disposal of rubbish will lead to increased fly and gnat breeding and the likelihood of a spread of diarrhoeal disease (p.102) and other infections.

If a family has little land for cultivation and is poor, parents will be unable to buy sufficient food for their families. This will especially apply to expensive nutritious items for their young children, so that malnutrition of various types is likely to occur, including shortage of calories and protein (p.65), of iron (p.83), or vitamin A (p.96).

Lastly, the level of education is important. Illiterate parents with little knowledge of the needs of their children are likely to feed them on the wrong foods, so that again malnutrition can occur. They will also tend to give their children dirty water and food, so that diarrhoea may result.

Poverty, with associated low levels of hygiene and education, does not produce any special 'tropical diseases', it just leads to diseases seen all over the world, only more commonly and in more severe forms. It is the main cause for the great amount of childhood disease in the tropics, so that its improvement is essential if children are to be healthy. Improved child health and nutrition depend more than anything else on government policies, which help to improve the availability of income, land, food and health (and other) services for the poor. Child health workers need to recognize this, and support such developments when they can.

Health services

The situation is often made more difficult by insufficient coverage by health services, due to lack of funds and, very often, to an overemphasis on expensive hospitals and physicians, in major cities. Modern services need to consist of a network reaching from urban hospitals to health centres to village primary health services (p.215), organized with community participation (p.244), with emphasis on prevention.

Climate

Only a very few diseases in children are due to the effect of climate alone, such as the rash of prickly heat (p.188). Other conditions are due to the fact that various insects that transmit disease can breed more easily in the tropics, for example the anopheline mosquitoes which carry malaria (p.117).

Customs

Some disease in children can be due to harmful customs (p.14), such as tetanus of the newborn (p.37) which can result from dressing the cord with cow dung, or diarrhoea which can follow the use of strong purgative herbal medicines in a young baby.

Inherited disease

Some diseases, which are inherited from parents, are more common in various parts of the tropics. In particular, sickle-cell anaemia (p.90) is much more frequent among African populations.

Effect of improved child health

A lowered death rate in childhood means an increased population, and more mouths to feed, to find employment for, and who will need health and other social services. In tropical regions (as anywhere), the aim should be 'not more, but better children', leading on to a healthier adult population. In all parts of the world, family spacing should be an important method of producing fewer, healthier, better-cared-for children. This can be difficult to introduce because large families are often desired to assist in farming, for bride price (or dowry), and because parents expect at least half of their children to die in the early years of life.

Family planning programmes can often be best introduced through maternal and child health services (pp.215 and 224); they can improve the health of both mothers and children, and the welfare, happiness and prosperity of families.

Closely spaced, over-large families affect the health of the mothers (p.6), as well as that of the children. Most importantly, parents become more willing to accept family planning when they know that most of their children will live rather than die. Child health services are, therefore, an important way to encourage parents to want to have smaller families and thus to appreciate advice on child spacing (p.217).

2
Maternal health and children

Kusum Shah

The health of mothers greatly influences the health, development and well-being of their children. The pattern of disease affecting children depends on the genetics (inherited conditions) and the environment. In childhood, both of these are very closely linked with the mother, yet in many developing countries the decision-makers in families do not give much importance to the health of women and their daughters, who are the future mothers. This preferential behaviour of a society can be a cause of ill health in children. Many diseases in children can be prevented and their growth and development improved if mothers are healthy from their own childhood, through pregnancy and breast-feeding, and if their knowledge, attitudes and practices are such as to benefit their own health and that of their children.

Maternal health before pregnancy

Some diseases are genetically transmitted to children from the mother (or father). Sickle-cell anaemia (p.90) is an important example in African communities.

Pre-pregnancy nutrition

The maternal nutrition before pregnancy has a strong influence not only on the growth of the fetus and birth weight of newborn, but also on nutrition during infancy. A well-nourished woman generally delivers a well-nourished baby, and she has an ample supply of milk providing adequate calories and other nutrients to the breast-fed child. Those women who have chronic malnutrition of long standing before pregnancy deliver low birth weight babies. Severe chronic malnutrition in women influences their ability to

6

produce sufficient breast milk (p.56). Proper nutrition of girls during their childhood is extremely important for the nutrition and health of their own children in the future. In particular, emphasis should be placed on the need for equal care of daughters and sons.

Infections prior to pregnancy

Maternal antibodies passed to the fetus through the placenta provide protection for some months after birth against some of the common infectious diseases. If mothers have had these infections many years ago, or have never had them, then their young infants are susceptible at an early age. It is better if a woman suffers from infections, especially rubella (German measles) in her childhood or any time before pregnancy; otherwise, if contracted during early pregnancy, it may affect the growing fetus and cause congenital deformities. Chronic infections like tuberculosis and leprosy, which are common in developing countries, are usually acquired by women much earlier than during pregnancy. Tuberculosis severely affects the nutritional status of women.

Maternal health during pregnancy and labour

The mother's nutrition and infections during pregnancy can greatly affect fetal growth.

Birth weight

Pregnant women who are well nourished, and gain about 8–10 kg weight, deliver babies having good birth weights. By contrast, severely malnourished women and those who put on very little weight during pregnancy deliver low birth weight infants (p.42). Improving the nutrition of severely malnourished pregnant women increases the birth weight of their newborn infants.

Moderately and severely anaemic pregnant women deliver

low birth weight babies, who have poor iron stores and may also develop anaemia during infancy. Oral iron (and in some areas folic acid) administration in pregnancy is recommended in moderately and severely anaemic women for their own well-being, as well as for that of their infants. Severely anaemic women may need higher doses of iron by mouth, or iron injections.

Infections during pregnancy and the child

Acute infections such as rubella (German measles), and possibly other viral diseases, can cause congenital deformities in the fetus or an abortion. Many other infections can pass from the pregnant women to her unborn child. In particular, syphilis in the mother can lead to congenital infection in the newborn baby. In some countries the commonest infection during pregnancy is malaria, which may lead to fetal death or low birth weight. (p.42).

Infection in the mother's birth canal can cause infection of the amniotic fluid surrounding the fetus in the uterus (amnionitis) or the placenta (placentitis), which can lead to intrauterine fetal death or low birth weight. The newborn can swallow the infected amniotic fluid and suffer from diarrhoea, pneumonia or septicaemia.

Tetanus neonatorum is one of the commonest causes of deaths in newborn babies in developing countries. Its presence and severity can be due to low levels of maternal antibodies against tetanus. In areas of high risk, women should receive tetanus toxoid during pregnancy, or earlier (p.164).

Chronic diseases during pregnancy and the child

Heart and kidney diseases, urinary tract infections and high blood pressure before and during pregnancy can lead to abortions, stillbirths, low birth weight and a high perinatal mortality. However, it is important that diseases during pregnancy be managed with drugs which are not harmful to the fetus.

Smoking and alcohol

Smoking and the use of alcohol during pregnancy adversely affect the future child and should not be continued. Smoking during pregnancy retards growth of the fetus and causes low birth weight in the newborn, and, with alcohol, can also lead to fetal deformities ('fetal alcohol syndrome').

Heavy work and stress

Heavy physical work during late pregnancy has been blamed for causing low birth weight while psychological stress, as can occur in teenage pregnancies, can have adverse effects on the fetus.

During the antenatal period, health protection of the fetus (and child) must be through the mother — by treatment or prevention of infections and diseases, by ensuring adequate nutrition and psychological security and, if possible, by attention to conditions of work.

Labour and the child

Healthy, well-nourished, non-anaemic women with an adequate-sized pelvis usually encounter no problems during labour. However, birth injury can be an important cause of neonatal deaths and illness, leading in severe cases to cerebral palsy, mental retardation and epilepsy. Antenatal supervision and careful obstetric attention are important.

Mother's health during lactation and the child

Breast-feeding is the best method of feeding during the first 2 years of life, provided other foods (multimixes, p.61) are introduced by the fourth to sixth months. The mother's milk not only provides all the nutrients needed for the rapid growth of the child, but also protects against various infections. Colostrum produced during the first few days of lactation is particularly beneficial in preventing infections.

The production of the breast-milk depends in part on the mother's health, as well as on breast-feeding reflexes (p.56). If she is very seriously ill or severely malnourished or anaemic, the amount of milk production is less than it could be. Oral contraceptives should be avoided as they interfere with milk production.

The mother's emotional situation is also important. If she has confidence, breast-feeding is likely to be successful (p.56). Sometimes, young mothers who have no previous experience of breast-feeding, as well as highly educated women from economically well-to-do families, are anxious and uncertain and develop lactation failure (p.56). Artificially fed infants have much greater risks of diarrhoea (p.102).

The local conditions of the breasts, such as a retracted nipples, breast engorgement, mastitis or breast abscess, can also lead to a lactation failure, and subsequent malnutrition in the infant. It is imperative that mothers are motivated, encouraged and advised concerning breast-feeding from early in pregnancy. If they are malnourished, attention should be given to improving their nutrition, by instruction and education (p.190) or by the issue of food supplements (p.235).

Post lactation period

Uncontrolled fertility drains the nutrition of the mothers, who become malnourished and anaemic. Their children become victims of a continuing cycle of extremely adverse situations created by large families which become malnourished, have repeated infections, and have limited opportunities for education and overall development. Planning of families is very important for the mothers as well as for the children.

Care of the mothers and children

The mother's health cannot be considered apart from that of the child. Hence, the health care of women during pregnancy, labour and the lactation period should always be an important part of primary health care; it is obviously coupled with the health care of children. However, mothers in many developing countries are not in a position to reach the health centre for a number of reasons, nor do they have much authority in making decisions in general or regarding their children. The approach for basic health care for mothers and children should centre round home visiting, which should be one of the highest priorities for primary health care workers (p.215).

3
Customs and child health

Derrick B. Jelliffe

All over the world people have developed different ways of living and behaving, and these customs are especially important to the health of mothers and their children.

Reasons for importance

1. In tropical countries, much disease in children is preventable by such large-scale methods as improved water supplies and sewage-disposal systems, immunization against certain infections (p.201) etc., by means of health education (p.190) and a fairer distribution of income and land.

Health education, which means persuading mothers (and fathers and other relatives) to feed, clothe, house and care for their children better in their own homes, can be carried out only if local customs, both good and bad, are known. In fact, health education consists of trying to discourage or modify bad customs while encouraging those that are good.

2. Mothers will accept advice more readily and have more confidence if it is given with a knowledge of local customs, such as how local foods are cooked and if the mother believes that certain of them are bad for children.

Groups of customs

Five groups of customs are particularly important to the health of children.

1. *Pregnancy and childbirth*. The foods eaten, the amount of work and rest allowed the mother, and other customs in pregnancy can affect the baby in the uterus. For example, in some places only a small amount of food is given in pregnancy in the belief that a small baby and an easy delivery

will result. This is harmful, as the infant will be born with a low birth weight, with poor food stores from the mother and possibly even with some brain damage.

At childbirth, the following customs may be important:

(a) *labour* — methods employed by birth attendant (i.e. positioning of mother during labour, local medicines used by mouth or in the birth canal, etc.);

(b) *newborn* — methods of handling at birth, when the child is put to the breast, etc.;

(c) *cord and placenta* — whether the cord is allowed to drain, how it is cut and dressed, and whether the placenta has to be buried or disposed of in a special way;

(d) *after birth* — diet and amount of rest for mother.

2. *Infant feeding.* Local methods must be known, including the customary length of breast-feeding, the first food introduced and when (with special reference to the use or avoidance of the more nutritious foods in the local diet). Mothers' *ideas* of foods must be known, such as suitable (or unsuitable) foods for infants, or those thought to produce disease, or those that must not be given during certain illnesses. If a local food has a very high place in people's minds (cultural superfood), this must be realized (i.e. rice in India). New habits (which may be harmful) must also be recognized, as, for example, the unnecessary use of the feeding bottle and expensive tinned milks for infant feeding (p.60), or the giving of costly aerated, bottled drinks, containing no nutrition, except sugar, with the increased risk of dental caries.

3. *Causes of disease.* Mothers may have quite different ideas as to what they believe to cause disease in their babies (i.e. evil spirits, witchcraft, eating forbidden foods, etc.) and it is important to understand their beliefs.

4. *Child rearing.* Local methods of bringing up children must be known, including how the child is separated from the breast (i.e. whether suddenly or slowly, whether the infant is sent away, etc.), the way children are disciplined, ceremonies at different stages of the child's life, and parents' ideas about when the child should be able to regulate his bowels.

Preferences for children of one or other sex (usually males) and practices towards different children need to be recognized (e.g. twins, breech births, those born with teeth or extra fingers).

5. *Women*. The health of children is much bound up with customs relating to women, including foods forbidden to them, especially during pregnancy and while breast-feeding (such as eggs, chicken, mutton and certain fish in parts of East Africa), and the position of the wife in the family, in particular whether she has any say in the amount of money available for buying foods for the children. Healthy, well-fed women, having equal responsibility with their husbands in stable homes are needed to produce and rear healthy children. Ideas concerning the ideal family size are also important.

Types of customs

Four types of custom will be found in all groups all over the world, including Western industrialized countries.

1. *Good* (beneficial), that is, likely to make children more healthy and to protect them from disease in the particular part of the world. Breast-feeding up to 2 years is a good custom in most tropical countries, provided other foods are also given to the infant from 4–6 months of age (p.61). Another good custom is the early feeding with fish 'tea' (or soup) in parts of Jamaica, and the 'chicken-a-day' diet recommended for women after delivery in many Chinese communities.

2. *Bad* (harmful), that is, likely to produce disease. The use of cow dung as a dressing for the cord is a bad custom as it easily leads to tetanus of the newborn (p.37). Others in various parts of the world are failure to give colostrum — the first breast-milk — (parts of Pakistan), severe food restriction and purgatives in the treatment of diarrhoea (parts of Latin America), female circumcision (Sudan), not tying the umbilical cord (parts of rural Uganda), and forbidding the feeding of fish to young children because it is believed to

cause worms (Malaya). Practices preventing ('blocking') the use of available foods, especially for pregnant women and young children, are called 'cultural blocks'.

3. *Unimportant.* These are customs which do not seem to have either good or bad effects on the child's health, such as, for example the heavy outlining of a baby's eyes with soot to keep off the 'evil eye' (India), or the delaying of hair-cutting until a child can talk (Jamaica). There is no need to do anything about these.

4. *Uncertain*, that is, when it is difficult to decide whether a custom is good or bad. For example, the use of various earths and clays by pregnant women (Africa and India) and the tight binding ('swaddling') of babies (Eastern Mediterranean).

Further consideration and new knowledge may alter ideas about customs. For example, chewing of an infant's food was at one time felt to be harmful, but would now be considered a good practice in many rural tropical areas. Also, the new use of lead preparations to outline baby's eyes, as in some Arab countries, means that this practice becomes harmful, as lead poisoning can occur.

Western customs

Customs in so-called Western countries can be put into similar groups. In particular, some practices in modern health services have become recognized as harmful (e.g. separating the newborn baby and the mother, unnecessary removal of the tonsils, and male circumcision, etc.). It is important not to adopt such harmful customs, or to stop them if they have been introduced.

Customs in an unfamiliar area

Anyone working in an unfamiliar area should try to find out as much as possible about local customs, as follows.

1. By enquiring from educated local people and from

foreigners who have lived in the country a long time (but realizing that they may not be well-informed about village practices), and by keeping one's eyes open and asking mothers about their ideas and customs.

2. By dividing the customs found into good, bad, unimportant, and uncertain.

3. By using the good customs in teaching mothers, by trying to change or modify bad customs by health education (p.190), by not troubling about unimportant customs, and by observing uncertain customs and deciding later to which group they belong. Ideally, health education and activities in health services should be a blend of beneficial practices from local tradition and Western customs.

4

Growth and development

F. John Bennett

Growth is an increase in size of the whole body or its parts, whereas development is an increase in skills and ability, as a result of increased complexity of the body's structures and formation, especially the central nervous system.

It is important to be able to measure growth and development. For the individual child, such measurement should be a routine part of diagnosis of the state of health, and it is also essential for estimating the child's progress. Measurements of growth of many children in a community can be used as an indication of level of nutrition, if they are suitably recorded and analysed. Growth and development are influenced by the following factors.

Nutrition

Growth and development can be seriously affected by lack of either sufficient or correct nutrients reaching the body. This can occur before birth due to poor maternal nutrition or placental conditions. It can occur after birth due to insufficient or incorrect feeding, diarrhoeal diseases or intestinal parasites interfering with absorption. Examples are the failure of growth seen in protein–energy malnutrition (p.65) and in roundworm infection (p.110).

Infections

Repeated severe or chronic infections interfere with nutrition and hence with growth. Infections, such as tuberculosis, whooping cough, diarrhoeal disease, measles, malaria, infestation with intestinal worms, lead to decreased intake (failure of appetite, vomiting, restriction of food by parents), increased losses through diarrhoea, blood loss, poor

17

absorption, raised temperature and increased needs.

Surroundings before birth

During pregnancy, the fetus may be injured or its growth retarded by many factors. If the injury occurs during the early months of pregnancy, various congenital abnormalities can result, such as malfunctions of, or damage to, the heart or special senses.

The following can harm and affect the baby's growth while in the uterus.

1. The mother's nutrition (see above), age (very young or old) or frequency of childbearing or short interval between births.

2. Mechanical injury.

3. X-rays.

4. Some virus infections in the first 3 months (e.g. rubella).

5. Untreated syphilis in the mother.

6. Insufficient oxygen reaching the fetus due to poor development or disease of the placenta.

7. Maternal malaria (especially affecting the placenta).

8. Certain drugs, e.g. alcohol, thalidomide and possibly some pesticides.

9. The mother smoking a great deal.

After birth

Children may vary in their ability to grow, but growth can be assisted by certain conditions. The socio-economic level is important and affects growth and development, because it determines (to a great extent) nutrition and food, money available, education, access to health services, housing, sanitation and water supply, all of which in turn influence the frequency and severity of infections. Poverty, on the other hand, retards growth and development because it is usually associated with all the above factors of malnutrition, repeated infections, large family size and social deprivation. Emotions can also influence nutrition and growth. Family disruption, as occurs in refugee situations, and separation of the child from the mother can be other causes of poor growth or even of growth failure.

Family size can influence growth: frequent and numerous babies in a family not only affect maternal health and nutrition, but also the amount of food available to each child, the duration of breast-feeding, and the amount of care given by the mother. Good growth also depends on all the systems of the body being healthy, so that severe liver, kidney, lung or heart disease or handicap such as cerebral palsy can prevent normal growth.

Heredity

Height, weight and rate of growth are often more alike in brothers and sisters than among unrelated persons. In certain families, rapid growth and early development are usual, while some children are small simply because their parents are small. The difference in size of children in different ethnic groups and countries may in part be inherited, but environmental factors such as nutrition and infection are more important determinants.

Growth of the fetus

Although the rate of growth of the baby in the uterus is very great, usually the needs of the fetus are provided for at the expense of the mother, but a very low iron, vitamin A or calcium content in the mother's diet in the last 3 months of pregnancy may lead to poor stores of these in the baby. If the pregnant woman's food is very poor in protein and calories, a low birth weight results and possibly damage to the brain of the fetus. A good diet for the mother produces a baby with a sufficient store of nutrients, makes less likely the complications in pregnancy, and preserves the mother's health so that the chances of living are increased for both mother and child.

At birth, the weight of the babies of well-fed mothers is in the region of 3 kg (6–7 lb) in most parts of the world. In the last month of pregnancy, fat is laid down and it is this which increases the birth weight. Babies in tropical regions have, on the whole, a birth weight lower than those born in more industrialized cold countries. The reasons for this include inherited racial differences, a poor diet in pregnancy, maternal infections, and malarial infection of the placenta. First babies in young mothers are usually smaller at birth than subsequent ones, and also twins are usually smaller at birth than single babies.

Birth weight of the baby is an index of the nutrition of the mother and of the care she received during pregnancy, so for a whole community it can be an indicator of maternal malnutrition and of maternal health services. This, however, requires health workers to record this measurement whenever possible, so that an average can be worked out and also the percentage of births under 2500 g can be calculated. During the first few days of the newborn period, some weight loss occurs due to the passing of urine and meconium, but this is usually less than 10 per cent.

Measurement of growth

The relationship of rate of growth to a child's health is well known, and by comparison of measurements of a child over a period of time with those of other healthy children, it is possible to tell if he is growing well. This is best done by marking the weight (and, if possible, the height) every 2–4 weeks on a graph on which is printed the normal growth curve prepared from the measurements of a large number of healthy children, preferably from the same part of the world. Graphing a child's height and weight in this way may bring to notice growth failure due to illness, malnutrition or other causes long before other signs occur and can be used in Young Child Clinics (p.224). Graphs of a child's growth can also be used for teaching mothers about nutrition. The *Road to Health Chart* is often used (p.227) and is very valuable.

The flattening of the growth curve commonly seen in children in the tropics between the ages of 6 months and 2 years is due to: (i) the child's high need for protein and calories not being satisfied by the diet provided — breast milk by itself is no longer sufficient; (ii) the higher incidence of intestinal worms as the child is now eating different, often contaminated, foods and playing in the family compound; (iii) more infections (diarrhoeal disease, malaria, whooping cough and tuberculosis), some of these following waning of immunity derived from the mother; and (iv) the arrival of another baby leading to psychological and other consequences (e.g. less attention) for the weaned child.

Body weight

When weighing a child, it is important to exclude errors due to clothing, oedema, anklets, etc. The best type of scale for clinical or community use for weighing young children is one which is strong, transportable and easy to use (p.230). Weighing is best done by workers who have all learned to do the procedure in the same way. Scales should be checked regularly. Weighing should be carried out at the centre, clinic or in the home at intervals to judge the adequacy of growth and to detect early malnutrition (p.227).

Approximate average weights for age which are useful to remember are:

birth	3.5 kg
6 months	7 kg
1 year	10 kg
2 years	12 kg
3 years	14 kg
4 years	16 kg
5 years	18 kg
6 years	20 kg

Average weight gains

First 3 months	30 g (1 oz) per day

First 6 months   0.5–1.0 kg (1–2 lb) per month
Birth weight doubled by 5–6 months
Then 0.35–0.5 kg (¾–1 lb) a month until end of first year
Birth weight tripled at end of first year
During second year, 0.25 (½ lb) a month
Then about 2 kg (4–5 lb) a year until 10 years, the gain being less regular

Body height

The international growth chart which is kept in some clinics has a graph (separate charts for boys and girls) for height. In infants under 2 years, length is measured supine on a special board, and in children over 2, height is measured standing. Height is useful for determining if a child is stunted or short for age, which may indicate long-standing malnutrition.

By comparing weight for height, it is also possible to show that a child is underweight, and this is useful when the age is not known.

However, in practice, few centres or clinics possess height or length boards.

Average heights (lengths) for age are:

birth	50 cm
6 months	65 cm
1 years	75 cm
2 years	85 cm
4 years	100 cm
6 years	113 cm

Average height gains

The body height is increased by 50 per cent at the end of the first year and it is doubled at the end of 4 years. The child's probable adult height may be estimated roughly by doubling the height at 2 years of age. Height of a child is particularly linked with parental height.

Puberty growth spurt

The alterations of body shape with growth from infancy to adulthood result from different rates of growth of various parts of the body at each stage of development. Variations of rates of growth also account for the differences in average size and shape seen between the sexes, and then become more marked in the second 10 years of life. During early adolescence, there is a rapid gain in weight which corresponds in both sexes to a gain in height. The rapid growth at adolescence occurs about 2 years earlier in girls than in boys. In general, the better the nutritional and social level of a child, the earlier the rapid growth of puberty begins and the sooner growth is completed. The stage of puberty is usually assessed in girls by development of the breasts and pubic hair and the onset of menstruation (menarche). In boys it is assessed by muscular development, changes in the voice, pubic and facial hair, changes in the size of the penis and testes, and emission of semen. As there is considerable variation between individuals, health workers must be prepared to explain this fact to anxious parents.

During the school years, the average normal gain in height is 5 cm. The rapid growth of adolescence in girls starts between 10 and 13 years. There is little increase in a girl's height after 16 years, and growth stops at about 18 years, depending partly on when menstruation started. In boys, the rapid growth of adolescence follows the same pattern as in girls but about 2 years later, so that growth ceases at approximately 20 years. In some parts of the world, due to prolonged malnutrition, puberty may be much delayed and slow growth continues for longer, even though the adults are short when it ceases.

Other important aspects of growth and development

Dental

The temporary teeth appear on average between 6 and 30

months. From 6–12 months the eight incisors first appear. The four premolars follow next between 12 and 18 months, and the four canines erupt between 16 and 22 months. The last four second premolars appear from 24–30 months. Up to the age of 2 years, a rough estimate of the baby's age may be gained by counting the number of teeth and adding 6 to give the age in months, e.g. a baby with 2 teeth is 2 + 6 = 8 months old.

The primary dentition starts to fall out at 6 years and this is completed between 10 and 12 years. The permanent teeth appear between the ages of 6 and 21 years. It is important to remember that the teeth are formed while the baby is in the uterus, so the mother's diet (and drugs such as tetracycline) affect their formation.

Head measurements

The circumference of the head (the greatest measurement just above the ears and round the forehead and the back of the head) at birth is about 35 cm ($\pm$ 1 cm). This increases by 1–2 cm monthly for the first 4 months, while a further 5 cm are added in the remaining 8 months. Thus the head increases in size by about 10–12 cm in the first year of life but after this, until the age of 20 years, it grows only another 10 cm. More rapid increase in size than this may be due to an abnormality, such as hydrocephalus.

Muscle growth

In early childhood, growth of muscle is very rapid and this is one of the reasons for the child's higher need of protein. A baby's upper arm circumference increases from about 10 cm at birth to about 16 cm at 12 months, but only by 1 cm in the next 4 years. In malnourished children, the small arm circumference is due especially to poor musculature.

Skeletal

Within a few months of birth, only the anterior fontanelle remains open, and this usually closes by 18 months.

Heart rate

It is important to remember that a baby's heart beats faster than an adult's. Usual average rates are as follows: birth, 140 per minute; first month, 130 per minute; 2–4 years, 100 per minute; 10–14 years, 80 per minute.

Development of immunity

This is a very important part of a child's development, and is discussed elsewhere (p.201).

Behaviour, social and mental development

The aspects of behaviour which develop as the child's central nervous system matures are posture, the combined use of the senses and muscles, speech and personal behaviour in society. All have patterns of development which differ in different countries, depending on the opportunities for practice and on the influence of the group culture (customs).

Simple records should be kept of milestones. Average times for babies in Europe and America are: holding up the head, 3 months; sitting supported, 6 months; sitting unsupported, 9 months; standing holding on, 10 months; standing unsupported, 13 months; walking alone, 15 months; few words at 1 year; short sentences at 2 years; control of bowels at 2½ years; control of urination at 3 years. However, there is considerable variation in these times, and in Africa, for example, babies are often much more advanced, even at birth, and can stand unsupported at 10 months and walk alone by 12 months. One of the reasons for this is that these babies are carried by the mother and played with more frequently so that their muscles and co-ordination develop more rapidly than if they were left for long hours in a cot.

Some reasons for a delay in development are ill-health (such as malnutrition), mental deficiency, or psychological causes, such as being separated from the mother. Delay in only one skill developing may be due to some deformity from birth, e.g. delayed walking due to congenital dislocation of the hip.

Social development as an accepted member of a society is usually aided by the parents and family. In the beginning, the mother is the main influence, but later increasing numbers of other people and experiences influence the child's personal behaviour. All children need a feeling of security and of being loved if they are to grow up into emotionally stable people.

Early childhood is a period of intense learning in which the physical, emotional, social, and knowledge and understanding elements are all closely linked. Many aspects of the environment can stimulate and help this learning and development in childhood. These include the important close link between mother and baby after birth, which is helped by breast-feeding, the type of stimulation given in the early years, e.g. from preschool and play opportunities, and the background of security provided by an intact and loving family.

5
The newborn

Olikoye Ransome-Kuti

A normal full-term newborn is one which is delivered after a period of pregnancy lasting 38 to 42 weeks (approximately 9 months). At birth, the baby weighs about 3 kg (6–7 lb) and cries loudly as soon as it is delivered. Breathing takes place immediately. The baby's colour is pink and he is able to move both arms and legs. The body may be covered with a sticky yellow substance called vernix, which protects the skin while in the womb. During the first days of life, a normal baby loses weight, but should regain the birth weight by the seventh to fourteenth day; this occurs earlier if the baby is breast-fed.

General care at birth

As soon as the baby is born, the following aspects of care should be attended to.

1. The mouth should be gently cleaned with a swab to remove any mucus which could be aspirated and prevent breathing.

2. Before cutting the cord, the baby is held horizontally below the level of the mother for about 1 minute, making sure that breathing has started satisfactorily. This will enable the baby to get extra blood from the placenta. Then the cord is tied with a sterile string in the usual manner and cut with a new razor blade or a sterile pair of scissors. Make sure that bleeding from the cord has stopped after it has been tied.

3. The eyes should be gently wiped with a swab and a few drops of 1% silver nitrate solution or freshly prepared penicillin eye-drops put into them.

4. The baby is handed over to the mother for her to carry and is permitted to suck on her breasts. This procedure improves the future relationship between the mother and the

27

baby, promotes contraction of the uterus and helps initiate breast-feeding.

5. The baby is placed in a cot near the mother or, if the bed is large enough, on the same bed as the mother, with the head down, and covered with a soft blanket. It is important to keep the baby warm at all times.

After completing the third stage of labour and when the mother has been made comfortable, the baby is given a general examination beside the mother as follows.

1. The baby is (a) weighed and the weight charted on *The Road to Health* card (p.230), and (b) examined for obvious congenital malformation. Note particularly those which can interfere with the child's health and feeding, e.g. cleft lip or palate, imperforate anus.

2. The umbilical stump is examined again for any bleeding and is re-tied if necessary. It is wise to paint the umbilical stump with an antibacterial preparation, such as triple dye (a mixture of gentian violet, brilliant green and proflavine). In the absence of triple dye, an antibiotic spray (a mixture of neomycin, bacitracin and polymyxin) may be used on the stump. Powder in any form is best avoided, and the cord is left exposed. Avoid bandaging around the abdomen as it may interfere with breathing and give rise to asphyxia.

3. Excess vernix and any blood on the baby's body is removed using a soft cloth soaked in lukewarm water. It is the practice in some communities to scrub the baby's skin with a rough sponge immediately after birth. This is to be discouraged. The baby should be allowed to recover from the process of birth for at least 24 hours before it is bathed. As a rough sponge may damage the skin, causing an opening for bacterial infection, a soft cloth, soap and lukewarm water should be used.

4. The baby should be clothed (and completely covered) with a light (cotton) garment to prevent loss of heat but allow him to move freely.

If the baby is wrapped, a cotton sheet should be used and the wrapping should be loose, again, to allow the baby free movement.

5. Vitamin K 0.5–1 mg should be given orally or intramuscularly to prevent bleeding during the first week of life.

Normal full-term baby

The aim is to establish breast-feeding in a normal full-term baby. The baby should be put to the breast as soon as he appears to be hungry. No other type of food should be offered. It is even more important for the baby to get the colostrum from the breast for protection of the intestine against infection. Mothers must be discouraged from expressing the colostrum and throwing it away, as is the harmful custom in some parts of the world.

During the first 2 weeks or so after birth, the baby may continue to cry after breast-feeding. The reason may be that the flow of milk has not been established. *After breast-feeding*, and when the breasts are empty, the baby can be given boiled water, preferably by cup and spoon, although this should be avoided. Cow's milk preparation should be avoided. Steps must be taken to ensure a good flow of mother's milk as soon as possible. At this time, many mothers need support and encouragement with breast-feeding.

Ill full-term baby

A baby who is severely ill after delivery and cannot feed (e.g. suck or swallow) may need to be tube-fed. This procedure is normally undertaken in a hospital. Mothers should be encouraged to express the breast milk completely and regularly, and this should be fed to the baby. In this way, the mother's breast milk will continue to flow, and the baby can resume breast-feeding as soon as he is well enough to do so. If the culture permits it, the mother may be encouraged to suckle another baby so as to keep the breast milk flowing while her baby is still ill.

Conditions in the mother

Engorged breasts

If the mother's breasts are engorged, the baby should continue to feed on the breast but more frequently. The mother may also hand-express some milk out of the breast between feeds. A mild analgesic such as aspirin or paracetamol may be given to the mother to relieve any pain. Failure to relieve engorgement may cause the breast to dry up or may lead to a breast abscess.

Tuberculous mother

If the mother has tuberculosis, the following steps should be taken.

1. If the tuberculosis is 'closed', i.e. there are no bacilli in the sputum, the baby is given isoniazid (INH) (20 mg per kg body weight) which is continued until he is weaned. During this period, the baby is left with the mother to breast-feed. At the same time, the mother is put on adequate antituberculosis therapy. After weaning, the baby's INH is stopped; 48 hours later, the baby is given bacillus Calmette–Guérin (BCG) vaccine.

2. If the mother's tuberculosis is 'open', i.e. bacilli are present in the sputum, the same procedure is followed as regards INH and BCG given to the baby, but the baby is brought to his mother for breast-feeding only until her tuberculosis is closed, i.e. there are no bacilli in the sputum which is usually not more than a week or two if she is on adequate antituberculous treatment. After this period, the baby can be left with the mother to be breast-fed.

Problems immediately after birth

The baby fails to breathe

1. If the baby does not breathe within 3 seconds or is blue

(cyanosed) after delivery, do not wait for a minute as described previously. Clamp and cut the cord immediately. Gently suck out the mucus in the nose, mouth and throat using a soft rubber or plastic mucus extractor; then tap the soles of the feet briskly. The baby should begin to breathe immediately after a few gasps.

2. If the duration of failure to breathe is longer than 1 or 2 minutes, start mouth-to-mouth breathing immediately as follows. Place a few layers of gauze over the baby's mouth, while the nostrils are held closed. Blow very gently into the baby's mouth, using the air in your mouth only. This is repeated about 15 times a minute. Watch the baby's chest all the time to make sure that enough air is used to produce slight expansion. Continue mouth-to-mouth respiration until the baby breathes and the pulse or heart rate is about 100 per minute. If oxygen is available, direct a stream of it through a funnel onto the baby's face so that, at the first gasp, he breathes in a lot of oxygen.

Cyanosis

After breathing is established, the baby may be found to be cyanosed (blue). This may be due to disease of the heart or lung or to brain damage.

In the case of the heart, it is probably a severe congenital defect and the baby needs expert attention. He will not improve in oxygen.

If the lung is the cause, the baby will continue to breathe rapidly with sucking-in (retraction) of the spaces between the ribs and movement of the nostrils. This can be caused by aspiration pneumonia or failure of the lungs to expand. Nurse the baby in oxygen and give antibiotics, crystalline penicillin 100 000 units/kg per day in two divided doses and streptomycin 20 mg/kg per day until the child improves.

If the cyanosis is due to brain damage during delivery, the baby will be limp and inactive, and will breathe slowly. Clear the airway and nurse in oxygen. If fits occur, give phenobarbitone 8–16 mg intramuscularly or by tube, and repeat 6–8-hourly until the fits are controlled. Continue to nurse in oxygen until the child has improved.

Pallor (pale baby)

Pallor soon after delivery may occur in a baby whose hands and feet are blue and whose body is pale. He may be feeling cold. The baby only needs to be covered with warm clothing. Oxygen will not improve the condition.   Pallor may also be due to bleeding in the brain following birth injury. In addition to pallor, the baby will be limp and inactive, and the pulse will be slow. Keep the child quiet and give phenobarbitone 8–16 mg per kg body weight 8-hourly orally. A bleeding umbilical cord may also cause pallor. The umbilicus should be checked regularly to prevent this accident. Pallor can also occur in a baby born to a mother with antepartum haemorrhage.

In all cases, a haemoglobin (Hb) estimation must be made, and the baby should be given a blood transfusion if the Hb is less than 10g/100 ml.

Fits

A convulsion in the newborn is commonly due to brain damage or low blood sugar (hypoglycaemia).

Convulsion due to brain damage should be treated with rest and phenobarbitone. Hypoglycaemia can be prevented in the majority of cases by feeding the baby as early as possible. It can be diagnosed using Dextrostix. If the blood sugar is less than 30 mg per cent, glucose drinks should be given using a cup and spoon. The blood sugar test should be repeated every 2 hours. If the fit persists and the blood sugar remains low for 24 hours, the baby should be referred for expert attention.

A jittery baby is often thought to have convulsions. Slight jitteriness is very common in babies and usually subsides within a few weeks without any ill-effect. If persistent and prolonged, it may be due to brain damage.

Constipation

All normal babies should have their bowels open and pass a dark greenish-black meconium stool within the first 24 hours of life. Failure to do so may mean that the baby has intestinal obstruction, in which case the following should be done.

1. Examine the anus to see if it is open or narrowed, or even closed.

2. Look out for signs of intestinal obstruction, which are abdominal distension and vomiting, particularly if the baby vomits bile. If present, the baby must be sent to hospital.

Never give purgatives, even in the mildest form, to a newborn.

Vomiting

Vomiting may occur in a newborn during the first 24 hours for the following reasons.

1. If he swallows meconium, blood or pus during delivery, causing irritation of the stomach. A bowel washout with 2 per cent solution of sodium bicarbonate or cooled boiled water should be done, and the vomiting should subside within 24 hours.

2. A congenital abnormality of the oesophagus may cause vomiting and aspiration distress with frothing in the mouth and nose immediately after the first feed. Feeding should be suspended and the baby referred immediately to hospital.

3. If there is intestinal obstruction, vomiting will be continuous or bile stained or projectile (leave the mouth forcefully). Other signs, such as constipation with or without abdominal distension, will be seen, and the baby should be referred to hospital.

4. Vomiting may also be due to overfeeding.

Problems after 24 hours

Infections

Newborn babies have no protection against many common infections caused by bacteria such as *Staphylococus, Esch. coli, Proteus vulgaris, Pseudomonas* and *Streptococcus*. These bacteria therefore cause many illnesses and death during this period. Every effort must be made to prevent these infections in the baby by general cleanliness during and after delivery, by breast-feeding, special care of the umbilicus, and keeping the baby away from adults with even a slight infection.

Skin infection

1. *Pemphigus*. This skin infection is caused by staphylococi or streptococci. It appears as blisters anywhere on the body, but may occur most around the neck or napkin area. The blisters at first contain clear fluid, which later becomes yellow in colour. When they burst, they leave red *inflamed* areas. The skin peels off in the area infected. The condition is highly contagious, especially to the babies. It may be found that the mother (or caring for or handling the baby) has a boil on her hands or parts of her body and that the infection was transmitted by her to the baby.

If in a hospital, the baby should be isolated and a swab of the contents of the blister sent to the laboratory. The baby should be treated with procaine penicillin 60 000 units daily for 5 days. The blisters can be snipped and then painted with triple dye or gentian violet (1 per cent). Contacts with boils should also be treated to prevent recurrence in the baby.

2. *Boils and abscesses* are also caused by staphylococci. These may need incision and drainage if large. Treatment is with crystalline penicillin injections, 100 000 units per kg body weight in two divided doses daily for 5 days.

Eye infection (ophthalmia neonatorum)

This is usually caused by gonococcus from the mother's birth canal. It can also be due to other bacteria. Pus is formed in the eyes, which may be very swollen. If untreated, it may led to blindness.

If the baby is in hospital, he should be isolated, and a swab of the eye discharge sent for bacteriological examination. Freshly prepared penicillin drops should be put into the eyes every 2 hours for 24 to 48 hours. In hospital, the mother can be of reliable assistance in this treatment. The baby is also put on a course of crystalline penicillin, 100 000 units per kg body weight daily in two divided doses.

Umbilical infection

Because bacteria grow easily in the umbilical cord, it is a common site of infection. In a hospital, the infection may spread to other babies. It is therefore important to treat the umbilicus of every baby in hospital with triple dye or an antibiotic spray.

Infection of the umbilicus may be localized or may spread to the liver or throughout the body by means of the bloodstream. It must therefore be treated vigorously with local applications of triple dye, or an antiobiotic spray containing a mixture of neomycin, bacitracin and polymyxin, together with daily injection of crystalline penicillin, 100 000 units/kg body weight in two divided doses daily, and streptomycin 20 mg/kg body weight daily for 5 days.

Respiratory infection

A baby with respiratory infection has cough, rapid (more than 60 breaths per minute) and difficult breathing with in-drawing of the spaces between the ribs, and may be cyanosed. In addition, there may be a raised temperature. Newborn babies develop pneumonia quickly.

Treatment is with antibiotics such as crystalline penicillin,

100 000 units/kg body weight daily in two divided doses, and streptomycin 20 mg/kg body weight daily. Oxygen, if available, should be used only if the baby is cyanosed.

Diarrhoea

In all normal babies, during the first 3 days, the stools should change in appearance from the dark green of meconium to the normal yellow appearance, and become soft with a sour smell. After the first day or two, a normal breast-fed newborn may pass one to five stools a day. Some pass a stool after every feed.

In the case of diarrhoea, the stools become very loose or watery, appear green and are frequent. The baby begins to lose weight and soon becomes dehydrated. Diarrhoea is not common in babies who are breast-fed.

In a hospital, newborn babies with diarrhoea must be separated from other babies as the infection may spread to them. Swab from the stool should be sent to the bacteriology laboratory for culture and sensitivity testing.

In all cases of diarrhoea in the newborn, breast-feeding must be continued or the baby given expressed breast-milk with cup and spoon. As soon as the diarrhoea is noticed, in addition to breast-feeding, the baby must be given oral rehydration solution (p.106) or half-strength Darrow's solution orally, as much as he will take for at least 24 hours or longer, if the diarrhoea continues. This is to prevent dehydration. Antibiotics may also be indicated.

Septicaemia

It is common for infection of any part of the baby to be spread throughout the body by the blood stream. This is because newborns have little resistance to infection. The infection may be in the skin, umbilicus, lung, or intestine. Often there are no obvious abnormal signs. However, the baby is found to be ill, lethargic, not thriving and may be jaundiced. In some cases the baby may be severely ill. It is important to suspect septicaemia in such cases, and to start treatment immediately with crystalline penicillin, 100 000 units/kg body weight in two divided doses daily, and streptomycin 40 mg/kg body weight daily. In a hospital, blood culture should be sent to the bacteriology laboratory before starting treatment.

Tetanus neonatorum

This disease is commonly caused by infection of the umbilical cord with the bacteria *Clostridium tetani*, at birth or soon after. This occurs when the cord is cut with infected materials, such as bamboo sticks or broken bottles, or when the cord is traditionally treated with cow dung. Traditional methods of delivering babies on to the floor in homes, and precipitate delivery on the roadside or in motor vehicles on the way to the hospital are situations in which tetanus can occur in the newborn.

The disease begins between the third and tenth day of life. At first the baby cannot suck the breast because of stiffness of the jaw muscles. Soon after, the baby begins to have spasms which, at first are few, but later become very frequent and may be continuous. Breathing is affected and the baby may become cyanosed. During the spasms, the hands are clenched into a fist, arms are flexed, the legs straightened and the back arched. The jaw is clenched and the lips drawn tightly into a type of smile.

The baby must be treated in hospital, although a few have been treated as out-patients when the disease is mild. Treatment aims at:

1. preventing spasms with phenobarbitone and diazepam (Valium) (in some cases, diazepam alone is adequate);
2. killing the *Clostridium tetani* and preventing respiratory diseases using crystalline penicillin, 100 000 units/kg body weight daily in two divided doses for 1 week;
3. neutralizing the tetanus toxin by giving antitetanus serum (ATS) 10 000 units once only on admission; the danger

of severe sensitivity must be avoided by prior tests ('sensitivity tests');

4. preventing the spasms by nursing in a quiet and dark area.

The baby must be tube-fed with the mother's expressed breast milk, using a nasal polythene catheter reaching into the stomach and kept in place until the baby is able to take feeds by mouth.

Tetanus neonatorum can be prevented by: (a) immunizing all pregnant women (or all older schoolgirls), (b) paying attention to cord hygiene at birth and until it drops off, and (c) giving ATS 750 units to all babies born on the floor at home, on the roadside, or in motor vehicles, before the disease appears. An important part of such a programme is the training of TBAs (traditional birth attendants).

Thrush

This is a common infection caused by a fungus. It occurs as white spots on the inside of the lips and cheeks, and also on the tongue. The spots may enlarge and join up to form a complete covering which is difficult to scrape off. Although the infection is not serious, it may spread to the intestine or the lungs. Treatment is by applying 1 per cent watery solution of gentian violet twice daily to the mouth until cured. It may also be treated with oral nystatin (Mycostatin) drops, 100 000 units three times a day for 5 days.

Haemorrhage

In some babies, between the second and eighth days, bleeding may occur from the umbilicus or the intestines, when the stool passed will be red or black. This is because the babies' blood is not able to clot properly. To correct this abnormality, such babies must be given an intramuscular injection of vitamin K, 1 mg. If the bleeding does not stop within 2 hours, the baby must be referred to hospital for possible blood transfusion. This should be given cautiously to avoid overload; often 20 ml of blood per kg body weight may be safely used.

Jaundice

In many tropical countries, jaundice in the newborn is a serious condition. When it is severe, it can cause brain damage or death. Slight jaundice which disappears in a few days, however, does not cause any illness in the baby.

In some cases, disease can be caused either by the lack of an enzyme in red blood cells or some differences in blood groups between the mother and the baby. These can lead to a destruction of red cells — and jaundice. The aim of treatment is to prevent brain damage by reducing the amount of jaundice-producing pigment (bilirubin) in the baby's blood. This can be done either by exchange blood transfusion or, to some extent, by exposing the baby to daylight. If the jaundice increases or the baby becomes ill and is unable to suck, he should be referred immediately for hospital treatment.

If jaundice occurs in a baby with umbilical infection and enlargement of the liver, it may be due to spread of a general infection (septicaemia) to the liver and should be treated with crystalline penicillin 100 000 units/kg body weight daily in two divided doses, and streptomycin 20 mg/kg body weight daily.

Jaundice accompanied by the passage of dark urine and pale stools may be due to abnormality of the bile ducts of the liver or virus infection of the liver (hepatitis). It may be one of the early signs of congenital syphilis. These babies should be referred to hospital.

Vomiting

Vomiting in the newborn should always be taken seriously. The babies must be referred to hospital if: (a) the vomiting is persistent; (b) it contains bile; (c) it is accompanied by constipation and/or abdominal distension.

Vomiting with loose stools suggests infective diarrhoea (p.102).

Breast enlargement

Milk-producing hormones passing from the mother to the baby during the last stages of pregnancy can cause enlargement of the breasts in some newborns. The enlarged breasts may produce milk, commonly called witch's milk. These settle down by themselves and should be left alone. They must not be squeezed as this may lead to infection.

Enlarged breasts in the newborn which are inflamed — that is, red, swollen and tender — are caused by infection. Treatment is with a 5-day course of crystalline penicillin 100 000 units/kg bodyweight daily given in two divided doses.

Birth injury

Occasionally, a baby may be injured in various ways during the birth process.

Cephalhaematoma

This is a rounded swelling on one side of the skull, appearing a few days after delivery. It is due to bleeding under the membrane (periosteum) covering one of the skull bones. No treatment is necessary. The mother should be reassured that it will disappear slowly after some weeks.

Fractures

The clavicle is the bone most frequently broken during delivery. A hard swelling appears on the clavicle some days after birth formed by the healing bone (callus). No treatment is necessary.

Other bones that may be fractured during delivery include the following.

1. Humerus: treat by bandaging the arm to the baby's side for 10 days. Be sure the bandage does not disturb breathing.

2. Femur: treat in a gallows splint.

3. Skull: depressed fracture must be referred to hospital immediately.

Nerve injuries

The nerves going to the muscles of the face (facial nerve) may be pressed in and damaged, especially if forceps are used. The baby will not move the affected side of the face. No treatment is needed and the weakness will slowly disappear.

The many big nerves (brachial plexus) running through the armpit (axilla) may be injured during delivery. The baby will not be able to move the affected arm, and should be referred to hospital immediately.

6
Low-birth-weight babies

Aaron Ifekwunigwe

Newborn babies should be classified by birth weight as well as by gestational age (length of time in the uterus), as both are important in identifying those infants at high risk of death and disease in the neonatal period. There are fairly reliable methods for the clinical assessment of gestational age when the date of the last normal menstrual period is not accurately known.

Definitions

The following have been approved by the World Health Organization.

Birth weight: the first weight of the fetus or newborn obtained after birth, preferably within the first hour of life.

Low birth weight (LBW): birth weight less than 2500 g (5½ lb).

The birth weight is influenced by many things including altitudes, nutritional status of the mother, and physique of the general population. Therefore, whenever possible, it is useful to work out a local practical weight standard suitable for the particular part of the world.

Gestational age: the duration of gestation is measured from the first day of the last normal menstrual period. Gestational age is expressed in completed days or completed weeks (e.g. events occurring 280 to 286 days after the onset of the last normal menstrual period are considered to have occurred at 40 weeks of gestation).

Small for gestational age (SGA) = small for date (SFD): denotes intrauterine growth retardation.

Pre-term: gestational age up to and less than 37 completed weeks (less than 259 days).

It should be mentioned that some authors suggested valid reasons for preferring 38 weeks (266 days) instead of 37.

Term: gestational age from 37 to less than 42 completed weeks (259 to 293 days).

Post-term: gestational age of 42 completed weeks or more (294 days or more).

The term *premature* is no longer recommended for newborns as it refers to termination of pregnancy before term.

Extent of the problem of low birth weight

No exact figures on the number of low-birth-weight babies are available, as information on birth weight is not generally reported by countries. However, the World Health Organization estimates the number to be about 22 million live-born, low-birth-weight babies per year, or 17 per cent of the total annual live births in the world.

The percentage of low-birth-weight babies in various populations in the world ranges from 3 to more than 45. It is also estimated that only about 5 per cent of all low-birth-weight babies in the world are born in developed countries, while the rest (about 21 million) are born in developing areas, and roughly 16 million of these are small-for-date babies.

Causes of low birth weight

In more highly developed countries, birth weight has been associated with many factors. These include gestational age, maternal height and weight, maternal age, parity (number of births), socio-economic status of family, educational level of parents, smoking, drug abuse, nutritional status of mother, and infections and other maternal illnesses in pregnancy.

The less developed countries, in addition to the above factors, have other conditions that are closely associated with low birth weight. They are protein–energy malnutrition, anaemias and infections in the pregnant woman, and unregulated fertility (too many and too closely spaced births), made worse by poverty, poor environmental sanitation and inadequate (or absent) health and social services.

Various studies have shown the influence of *maternal nutritional status*, both before and during pregnancy, on the birth weight of the infant. The mothers who were well nourished before pregnancy and/or ate sufficient extra calories during pregnancy had children of both a higher average birth weight and a lower proportion of low birth weight, when compared with those who did not.

Anaemia of pregnancy, with haemoglobin values below 10 g/100 ml, is frequent in all parts of the world, but much more so in the less developed countries. Iron-containing foods etc. may be limited in the general diet and may be further restricted for women by custom (p.12). In addition, all women have higher iron requirements during the child-bearing age, further increased by the extra demands for iron and folates during repeated pregnancies. The low oxygen in the anaemic mother's blood would interfere with the growth of the fetus.

The *infection of mothers during pregnancy* with some viruses, especially rubella (German measles) and bacterial infections of the urinary tract, are well known to be associated with low birth weight. There is also some evidence that illness during pregnancy is associated with low birth weight. Of great importance is the role of *malaria*. This applies not only to clinical malaria, but also to the quite common malarial infection of the placenta, which is usually without symptoms. Control of malaria and/or prevention with antimalarials during pregnancy lead to increased birth weight.

Short intervals between birth due to *unregulated fertility*, are associated with low birth weight. This is presumably due to the using up of maternal stores resulting from the lack of a sufficient interval for recuperation between pregnancies.

In fact, low birth weight and socio-economic conditions in any population are so strongly related that birth-weight distribution and proportion of low birth weight have been suggested as good indicators of socio-economic development in that population.

Assessment of gestational age at birth

The obstetrician uses various methods to estimate the gestational age of the fetus. Most simply, these include the date of the last normal menstrual period, size of the uterus and fetus, time of fetal movement, and time of detection of the fetal heart sounds with the fetal stethoscope.

After birth, the physical characteristics and state of development of the nervous system (neurological assessment) are used for estimating gestational age. However, neurological assessment is unreliable if the infant has a central nervous system disorder, such as cerebral haemorrhage, or if the mother has been anaesthetized.

The gestation of a baby can be adequately estimated in the first hour after birth, with a minimum of handling of the infant, by an experienced physician.

Risks of low birth weight

The increased risks of low birth weight are mainly due to the baby's lack of maturity. The following are some important examples.

1. Weak suckling, swallowing, gag, and cough reflexes, leading to difficulty in feeding and danger of aspiration of milk into the lungs.

2. Immature lungs and a soft chest wall, leading to breathing difficulties.

3. Decreased ability to maintain a steady normal body temperature.

4. Immature kidneys with limited ability to excrete waste products in the urine.

5. Increased susceptibility to infections.

6. Limited iron stores and rapid growth, leading to later anaemia (p.83).

7. Tendency to develop rickets due to rapid growth with diminished intake of calcium and vitamin D.

Management of the low-birth-weight infant

General

Routine methods applied to full-term infants should be followed. The umbilical cord should be tied with a double ligature with a narrow cotton tape about 6 cm from the abdomen (to allow for the possibility of exchange transfusion). No dressing is needed. All low-birth-weight infants should be given 1 mg vitamin K_1, by intramuscular injection, in order to prevent haemorrhage.

Low-birth-weight infants should be allowed to rest in their cots as much as possible, with a minimum of handling. They should be placed in the special care nursery or in incubators, if available, as soon after delivery as possible. However, feeding should not be delayed, because of the need for rest, for longer than 3–6 hours due to the risk of starvation and dehydration.

Warmth and humidity

Very low-birth-weight infants should be loosely clad in special flannelette gowns, and exposed as little as possible, especially at night. In hospitals without special equipment, they should be warmed by two to four hot-water bottles, filled with one-half hot and one-half cold water. These are fitted into a hot-water bottle cover of blanket material and placed in two canvas pockets at both sides of the cot, or placed under the cot. One of the bottles must be changed hourly. *Great care must be taken to follow instructions carefully, as otherwise burns can easily occur.*

Humidity can be raised in the special care nursery by means of a water sterilizer in the corner of the room or by a steam kettle.

Room temperature can be read on a wall thermometer. If it reads 29°C (85°F) or below, the heater will be put on; if above, it will be turned off.

Of course, when available, the infant is best placed in an

incubator. The incubator temperature should be kept high enough to maintain the baby's body temperature at 36–37°C (96.8–98.6°F). This is usually an air temperature of about 32–36°C (90–97°F) depending on the baby's size and maturity. The relative humidity is maintained at 40–60 per cent.

Rectal temperatures should be taken at least twice a day with a low-reading thermometer. If raised above 37°C (99°F) or below 35.5°C (96°F), the temperature should be taken 4-hourly, and the doctor notified.

Oxygen administration

Infants who suffer from respiratory distress become deprived of oxygen (hypoxic) and cyanosed (blue). They should be given oxygen, and a simple form of oxygen tent can be prepared from old x-ray films, in the form of a five-sided box with a perforated top, which can be placed over the baby. The oxygen is led into the box through a rubber tube introduced low down on one side of the box.

Warning: No naked flame to be exposed near oxygen to avoid risk of fire.

Control of infection

The following measures will help to control infections.

1. Infants should receive breast milk (including colostrum, p.54) whenever possible.

2. All infected staff (i.e. with skin infections, boils, 'cold', diarrhoea, etc.) should be kept out of the special care nursery.

3. No relatives, except mothers, should be allowed in.

4. All infants with infections should be isolated in special cubicles.

5. Frequently changed double-layer masks may be worn by staff, if feasible.

6. Frequent handwashing by staff, especially between handling babies, and by mothers, especially before feeding their infants, is important.

7. Infants born more than 12 hours prior to arriving at hospital should be admitted in an isolation cubicle and given a course of antibacterial therapy.

8. After discharge, sheets are washed and blankets 'sunned' or, preferably, autoclaved. If the cot is made of canvas, it should be thoroughly washed and 'sunned', or, if metal, it can be carbolized.

Feeding

Time of commencement

Early feeding, even in very low-birth-weight infants, is preferred to periods of starvation and dehydration. Feeding should be started as soon as the infant has recovered from birth, approximately 3 to 6 hours after birth, in those without complications.

Type of feed

Breast-feeding is essential for survival of the infant in most situations in developing countries. If suckling at the mother's breast is not possible, expressed breast milk (EBM) is given, and this should be expressed by the mothers before each feeding time. It is important that mothers express *all* their breast milk before each feed, *in order to maintain lactation*. Breast milk, if not used for that particular infant, can be thrown away, or properly refrigerated or boiled and saved for use on another infant.

If EBM is not available at all, or in insufficient quantity, complete or complementary feeds could be prepared from a reliable, economical, locally available half-cream, powdered cow's milk preparation, fortified with vitamin D and iron. Feeds can be prepared by adding 1 measure (or level teaspoonful) of powder to 30 ml (1 fl oz)* of cooled boiled water, with the addition of 30 g (1 oz) sugar to 560 ml (1 pint) of mixture to increase the calories. It is vital that the strictest attention be paid to hygiene in the preparation of feeds.

Quantities

A first feed of 4 ml (1 drachm) sterile water can be given to test the swallowing reflex. This can be followed by total daily amounts of about 15 ml (4 teaspoonfuls) of *expressed breast-milk per kg birth weight per day of age*, divided into seven 3-hourly feeds. The feeds are increased gradually until the baby is receiving 160 ml or more per kg body weight (3 fl oz per lb) per day, which supplies about 120 kcal (504 kJ) per kg body weight or more.

Method of feeding

The method depends on the ability of the infant to suckle and swallow, and is usually related to the size of baby and whether there are any complications. If he can suckle and swallow, he can be fed on the breast or with the Belcroy feeder, which is a small-sized feeding bottle suitable for the infant's small mouth. If he can swallow, but is unable to suckle, a spoon or rubber-tipped pipette can be employed. Finally, if he can neither suckle nor swallow, feeds must be given via a nasogastric polythene tube, or, in very sick infants, where possible, intravenous feeding of 10 per cent glucose may be necessary. As the infant becomes more mature, so the method of feeding changes, ultimately aiming at his being breast-fed.

Feeds by modified Belcroy feeder, pipette or spoon can be administered by mothers, after they have been shown the method. Care must be taken that they wear masks and wash their hands.

*Conversions from ounces and drachms to ml. are given in practical approximations.

Test of feeding ability

In all cases, the first feed of sterile water can be started carefully, using a spoon to test the particular baby's ability to swallow.

Test of growth

Very low-birth-weight infants can be weighed twice weekly, while the bigger infants can be weighed daily.

Position after feed

The infant should be placed on his right side with the head slightly elevated for about half an hour. This helps to prevent regurgitation of feed, with the danger of inhalation into the lung.

Follow-up

The infant should be given supplements of polyvitamin and iron. When the infant has progressed and grown enough, and the mother has been adequately trained to care for him, he can be discharged home.

Every effort must be made to ensure that the baby is being breast-fed on return home. If he is not, there is little chance of his surviving. If no breast milk is available, the preparation and use of cow's milk feeds, stressing cleanliness with regard to feeding utensils, must be repeatedly shown to the mother, who must herself carry out the procedure under supervision. The most economical, reliably, locally available full-cream milk powder can be used, or good quality fresh milk, if available, which must be bought and boiled each day.

If fresh milk is used, 3 parts boiled milk is added to 1 part of water. A similar mixture can be prepared by adding 15 measures (or level teaspoonfuls) to 560 ml (1 pint) of water. About 180 ml per kg body weight (3 fl oz per lb) per day should be given. Instructions may be given to add sugar, 30 g to 560 ml (1 oz to the pint), to either of these mixtures, to increase the calorie content, if the mother is considered able to follow these more complicated instructions.

The mother must be shown how to make up feeds and must prepare them under supervision. She must be taught to use a cup and spoon, or a feeding cup, and must know how to keep them clean. A feeding bottle is not recommended for uneducated mothers because of the danger of infective diarrhoea.

If practicable, these infants must be followed up as out-patients for a long period. This is because of the high incidence of serious handicaps occurring later: cerebral palsy, deafness, learning problems and mental retardation. Early recognition of these and appropriate treatment are indicated, when feasible and available.

Prevention of low birth weight

The association between low birth weight and socio-economic status indicates that the ultimate solution to this problem of low birth weight will result from socio-economic development, including appropriate health care. In the short term, some measures need to be taken to reduce the size of this problem, especially the prevention of maternal malnutrition and illness during pregnancy, including infections (p.6). In between pregnancies, special attention should be paid to prenatal care, and the effective practice of family planning leading to child spacing, improved general health and nutritional status.

7
Young child feeding

Derrick B. Jelliffe and E.F. Patrice Jelliffe

Malnutrition in early childhood is common in many developing countries (p.65), so that ensuring the best possible feeding for young children is an important part of the health services everywhere (p.201). Attention needs to be given to: (1) the unborn child (the fetus), (2) the young infant (0–6 months), and (3) the older infant (6–12 months) and the 'preschool age' child (1–4 years). It is important to recognize that all stages are of importance and related to one another. For example, some malnutrition in later infancy can, in part, be due to fetal malnutrition, having given rise to a low-birth-weight newborn with poor nutritional stores.

Fetus

For 9 months, the unborn child (fetus) is 'fed' by the mother through the placenta and umbilical cord. Low birth weight (p.42) can be the result of many different causes, including, for example, smoking in pregnancy, high altitude, etc. In developing countries, however, infections in the mother during pregnancy, particularly malarial infection of the placenta, are important causes. In addition, poor maternal nutrition, often associated with infections as well, can lead to a low-birth-weight baby with poor stores of calories in the form of subcutaneous fat and of vitamin A, iron, etc. in the liver.

Fetal growth and nutrition cannot usually be measured directly without very special apparatus. However, measurements of the mother in pregnancy can indicate those at risk of giving birth to a low-weight newborn, for example a poor weight gain, a low weight for height, and a less-than-normal arm circumference (p.190).

Nutrition education (p.190) is always required to ensure

52

that the mother makes the best use of locally available foods during pregnancy. In addition, extra nutrients are required and can be looked up in the RDA (*Recommended Dietary Allowance*) used in the particular country. These can be then considered in terms of locally available food stuffs. Difficulties may occur with regard to obtaining a good diet during pregnancy as there may be a variety of cultural dietary restrictions on the type or quantity of food eaten at that time (p.12). Also, continuing hard work and poverty are often important.

Observation in a prenatal clinic or by home visiting during pregnancy is important for the mother's health and for a safe delivery. In addition, observation can be undertaken by weighing at intervals or measuring the arm circumference (p.96). Also, some clinical signs may need to be watched out for — in particular, a pale conjunctiva, usually as an indicator of iron deficiency anaemia (p.83). In some countries where a particular deficiency is common, other clinical signs may be specially important. For example, in Indonesia, the presence of Bitot's spots needs watching out for as these indicate vitamin A deficiency (p.96).

The use of food or nutrient supplements in pregnancy will vary with the particular circumstances and problems. In many parts of the world, iron tablets (ferrous sulphate) may be given to all mothers throughout pregnancy, or during the last 3 months, or to selected mothers with pale conjunctivas or low haemoglobin (p.96). In other countries, it may be desirable to give other nutrient supplements to selected mothers in pregnancy. For example, in areas where vitamin D deficiency is common, oral dosage of vitamin D may be advisable in pregnancy and during breast-feeding.

Food supplements may be available from international aid or, in a few countries, may be processed nationally or using simple technology at regional or provincial levels. The use of such supplements needs very careful consideration, but may be indicated especially in mothers who are showing signs of poor weight gain in pregnancy or a decreasing arm circumference. Problems with the supply of such supplements include cost, difficulties of distribution and selection, and, particularly with pregnant women, the likelihood that supplements distributed to them will, in fact, be given to the other members of the family as well.

Another, often under-appreciated, reason for trying to ensure a good weight gain in pregnancy is that under normal circumstances a mother lays down about 8 lb (4 kg) of subcutaneous fat during this period of time. This subsequently acts as a calorie bank for the first 3 months or so of milk production during breast feeding.

The young infant

In traditional circumstances, the young infant in the first 6 months or so of life has the same close contact dependence on the mother as the fetus in the uterus. For this reason, the young infant has sometimes been called the 'external fetus' with the mother's breasts taking the place of the placenta.

The breast-fed young infant

Breast-feeding with human milk has overwhelming advantages anywhere in the world, but especially in developing countries, where hygiene is poor and some families cannot afford to buy sufficient animal milk or formula and have inadequate education to be able to use these properly.

Human milk is exactly right nutritionally for the young infant's needs and, even in less than well-nourished women, supports growth by itself for some 4–6 months. Human milk also has a protective effect against infections, especially those leading to diarrhoeal disease. This is not only because it is clean, but also because it contains protective substances and white cells (especially in colostrum, the first yellowish milk produced after delivery). Breast-feeding also is the most ancient method of child spacing, provided the baby is taking the breast as required throughout the 24 hours, when it causes the menstrual periods to stop ('lactation amenhorroea').

Also, the contact between the mother and the baby during nursing is quite different and closer than when the baby is bottle-fed. This can lead to the loving link ('bonding') between the mother and the baby. Lastly, from a family and from a national point of view, breast-feeding has economic advantages. For the mother it requires only that she eats some more of the foods of her regular diet, whereas the use of animal milk or particular formulae means implementation from other countries, with the spending of foreign currency and with loss of an available food — that is, breast milk.

The length of time of breast-feeding advised depends on local circumstances. In traditional societies, this is usually for 2 to 3 years, or until the next pregnancy. Under natural circumstances, human milk is the *food for the first 4–6 months* and after this there comes the *supplement* (which, although small, is still of considerable importance nutritionally) to other foods in the diet.

Successful breast-feeding depends on two considerations — reflexes of the baby and mother, and maternal health.

During breast-feeding, the baby has three reflexes: the 'rooting reflex' (in which contact with the side of the baby's face leads to turning of the head towards this contact and opening and shutting of the mouth); the sucking reflex (in which the baby milks the mother's breast by pressing the end of it with his tongue against his hard palate; and the swallowing reflex. Usually in healthy, full-term babies these reflexes are present; however, if a baby is suffering from brain damage, severe jaundice, or severe infection at birth (septicaemia, p.36), then these reflexes may not be active. Also in premature (pre-term) babies, the reflexes are not yet active, so that it will be necesssary to feed the baby by intragastric tube-feeds (p.49).

In breast-feeding there are two maternal reflexes: the prolactin reflex and the let-down reflex. In the prolactin reflex (Fig. 7.1) the baby sucks the breasts, impulses pass on to nerves and to the pituitary gland in the brain, and the hormone prolactin is secreted into the blood and carried back to the breast, where it leads to the production of milk. The

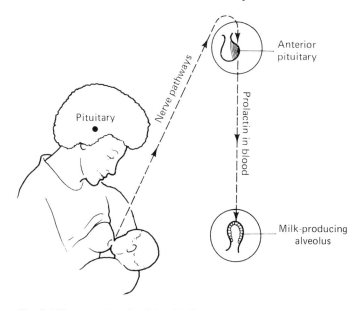

Fig. 7.1 The prolactin reflex (simplified).

let-down reflex (Fig. 7.2) is similar in that the baby stimulating the breast leads to nerve impulses to the posterior pituitary and the production of another hormone, oxytocin, which passes back to the breast and acts on small muscle cells which surround the sacks (alveoli) in which milk has been secreted. However, the let-down reflex differs from the prolactin reflex in that it can be interfered with by anxiety (e.g. "too little milk", "milk too thin") and can be made more effective by confidence. This means that anything which interferes with the mother's confidence can lead to interference with breast-feeding ('anxiety-nursing failure', Fig. 7.3).

The mother's health, including infectious diseases (such as malaria, tuberculosis, etc.), can interfere with lactation, as can severe maternal malnutrition. However, on the whole,

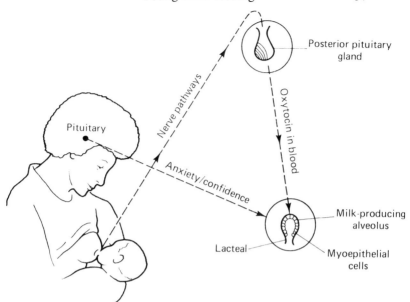

Fig. 7.2 The 'let-down' reflex (simplified).

less than well-nourished women breast-feed remarkably well, often at their own nutritional expense, However, in very poorly nourished women, the volume of milk produced is less than it could be, while if the mother is lacking in some nutrients, such as vitamin A, this can be reflected in lower levels in the milk.

In recent years, much progress has been made in understanding what is needed to promote successful breast-feeding. In general, information and education are needed for a wide variety of different individuals, including policy makers (relating to the economic aspects of loss of human milk), medical, nursing and nutritional professionals, schoolchildren and parents. The modifications in the management of the newborn baby can easily be made both in the maternity ward and on return home to ensure that the

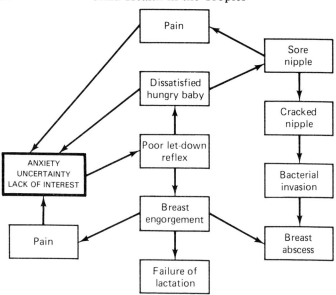

Fig. 7.3 Factors responsible for inhibition of the let-down reflex and lactation failure.

maternal reflexes are not interfered with. This means, in practice, early breast-feeding within the shortest possible time after delivery, the close contact between mother and newborn, and very frequent feedings as required by the baby during the 24 hours.

Health services for mothers must also be regarded as a part of any programme to promote breast-feeding, with methods of observing mothers in the prenatal clinic for poor weight gain during pregnancy, examination of the breasts (especially the nipples, p.22), and for the supply of food supplements for such mothers, if indicated and practical. Attention to mothers during pregnancy and breast-feeding is increasingly recognized as being of the greatest importance. Assistance is already given in most traditional societies, but, in urban communities which have become 'westernized,' there may be no female relative and/or traditional midwife to give physical and emotional support and to supply confidence and information. Under these circumstances, in many parts of the world such as the USA, UK, Scandinavia and Australia, women's support groups have grown up and their methods have been extremely successful.* In some countries, such as Brazil, such groups are rapidly developing in poor slum areas.

Programmes also have to take into account the special needs of working women, especially those in urban areas who may be going out to work in the labour force in factories, etc. The number of such women varies very considerably from place to place. In some countries, laws have been made which permit such mothers to have 'lactation leave' and/or to be able to take the babies with them to work, with crêches provided for them to leave their babies and to breast-feed several times a day.

Lastly, much attention has recently been given to the widespread promotion of infant formulae and developing countries by the food industry. It is now recognized that this needs to be controlled and a WHO Code of Marketing of Breast Milk Substitutes has been developed for guidance of all governments.

It is important that health workers of all levels appreciate the importance of *all* of these different measures to promote breast-feeding, which represent not only many positive advantages, but also which, if declining, can lead to an increase in disease in the form of marasmus (p.69) and diarrhoea (p.102), an increase in the birth rate and population pressure and an increased expenditure of foreign currency to import infant formulae from abroad.

The non-breast-fed young infant

In all countries, there will usually be a very small percentage

*The largest group is the La Leche League International (LLLI), from which information can be obtained: 9616 Minneapolis Avenue, Franklin Park, Illinois 60131, USA.

of babies who cannot be breast-fed. For example mothers may have died in childbirth, may have abandoned the babies or may have to work in jobs which make breast-feeding impossible. Alternatives to breast-feeding fall into two categories.

1. *Lactating women*. Depending on the culture, a lactating relative or a wet-nurse may be used. In some communities, lactation is started in a non-lactating woman by frequent sucking on the breast.

2. *Animal milk*. Sometimes a reliable source of animal milk may be available, (e.g. cow, buffalo, goat, etc.). Although quite different from breast-milk, cow's milk can be best modified by boiling, diluting with boiled water (2:1) and adding sugar (Table 7.1). Similarly, unsweetened evaporated milk or powdered full-cream cow's milk can be used, after initial dilution to the strength of basic cow's milk. Numerous 'modified formulas' are widely available, but are very expensive.

Whatever is fed to the non-breast-fed baby is extremely dangerous because of the likelihood of overdilution and bacterial contamination. The feeding bottle is especially risky as it is very difficult to clean. Although more difficult to use, a cup and spoon or feeding cup is much safer.

Table 7.1 Simplified use of cow's milk and its preparation in the feeding of babies up to 3 months of age

	Fresh cow's milk	Full-cream powdered milk	Evaporated milk
Dilution	2 parts boiled milk + 1 part boiled water	1 level teaspoon milk powder + 1 fl oz (28 ml) boiled water	1 part evaporated milk + 2 parts boiled water
Add sugar	1 level teaspoon household sugar per feeding		
Calculate daily volume	2½ fl oz per lb (140 ml/kg) body weight per day		
Calculate volume per feed	One-fifth of daily total at each of five feedings at 4-hourly intervals		

Weaning

Home prepared weaning multimixes

As the infant grows, other foods than breast milk need to be introduced by from 4–6 months. Such weaning foods should be based on the local staple ('cultural superfood') (p.13), together with other foods which together give all the nutrients that the rapidly growing young child needs. The high need for calories during this period, as well as protein, vitamins and iron, has been recognized in recent years. This need can be met by trying to ensure more frequent meals than are often usual for adults (e.g. four to five each day), by making the porridges, pastes, etc. that the child receives as thick as possible, and by trying to add 'compact calories' (such as oil and fat), whenever possible. This need is understandable in light of the child's high energy requirements, and also because of his comparatively small stomach capacity. Home-prepared weaning foods should be made from locally available foods, should be acceptable to the parents' cultural beliefs and practices (p.12), low in cost, low in bulk, digestible, prepared without too much difficulty and contain *all* the nutrients required for growth during this period. Sometimes a special weaning 'multimix' may be prepared for the young child alone. However, more usually, such multimixes have to be prepared from the foods which have been cooked for the rest of the family or from the family pot. This becomes particularly necessary because of the cost of fuel and because of the very limited time available to the mother.

Two main types of staple foods are eaten throughout the world: *cereal grains*, such as rice, wheat, corn (maize) etc., and *non-cereal grain staples*, such as tubers and roots (e.g. potatoes, yams, etc.) and plantains. Of these, the cereal grain staples are preferable, but the value of non-cereal grain staples has been underestimated. This is because the nutritional value of the cereal grain staple is acquired while they are dry, and the non-cereal grain staples are in a much more moist and watery condition under natural

Table 7.2 Approximate protein content and amino acid deficiency of main categories of vegetable foods used in multimixes

Type of food	Protein (approx. %)	Amino acid deficiency
Cereal grain	≥10	Lacking in lysine
Legumes*	≥20	Lacking in methionine
Dark green leafy vegetables‡	4–10	Lacking in methionine

* Soya beans   40%.
‡ Dried: 30%.

Table 7.3 Village-level cereal grain multimixes*

	Ingredients
Double mix	Staple + legume
	or
	Staple + animal protein‡
	or
	Staple + dark green leafy vegetable (DGLV)
Triple mix	Staple + legume + animal protein
	or
	Staple + legume + DGLV
	or
	Staple + DGLV + animal protein
Quadrimix	Staple + legume + DGLV + animal protein

* Preferably with added compact calories (oil) and continued breast feeding.
‡ Mixtures with animal protein preferable in all mixes.

circumstances. During cooking, for example, rice absorbs two to three times its weight in water, whereas the boiled potato or sweet potato does not.

Such weaning multimixes can contain two to five different main types of food: the staple together with a legume (pea or bean), animal product,* dark green leafy vegetables (DGLV) and 'compact calories' (fat).

*The term animal product is used here because foods such as meat, fish, eggs and milk are *mainly* made up of protein containing all the essential amino acids which cannot be made by the body, *but*, at the same time, also contain fat and carbohydrates.

The way in which such mixtures can be made is shown in Tables 7.2 and 7.3. Such multimixes can also be made with non-cereal grain staples, but it is probably desirable to add animal products to such mixtures, even more so than with the cereal grain staples.

Processed weaning multimixes

In some developing countries, especially in the major cities, imported infant foods may be available in stores, shops and supermarkets. These include, for example, the glass jar foods so popular in America and Europe. However, it is rarely advisable for these foods to be used in developing countries. They are convenient and have the prestige of the purchased over the home prepared, but they are extremely expensive, relatively low in nutrients and are used in Western countries as *one* type of food in a mixture of others. In some developing countries these foods have been used, and in some cases the less expensive and less nutritious of them (e.g. apple purée) have been given alone — as though they were the only food required.

Special food mixtures

Special food mixtures, particularly designed for young children, have been manufactured in numerous countries over the past few decades. They have usually failed because they have not been able to compete successfully from a commercial point of view as their cost, although lower, is still higher than the basic staple which the mother will buy in preference. Also, various special weaning food multimixes have been imported from abroad as a part of aid programmes, including CSM (Corn Soy Milk) and WSB (Wheat Soy Blend). These can be extremely helpful, especially in emergency situations such as famines or refugee relief. However, these do not solve the problems on a long-term basis and, in any case, have to be associated with nutrition education activities, otherwise the danger is that the countries and families become dependent, and when, as can happen, supplies are discontinued, the original problem, far from being solved, has become worse.

In recent years, some countries have manufactured weaning multimixes locally using simple technology. These are made in the country or province concerned and contain a limited number of low-cost, locally available, culturally acceptable foods. They can, therefore, be used for nutrition education purposes. In the Phillipines and Burma, for example, these are now available in plastic packets which are subdivided so that the actual *ingredients* are present separately. The idea is that rather than an unknown powder made up of a mixture of ingredients, having them visible can provide direct evidence for the mother of the benefit of these foods, which she can be encouraged to purchase later. These educational multi-item packets are available at very low cost in stores, and, in some cases, free through government services.

Conclusion

'Young child feeding' has to be seen as a continuous process starting with the fetus in pregnancy, then the young infant and breast-feeding, and the older infant and the preschool-aged child with home-prepared weaning multimixes, together with a continuing, small but still important, supply of breast-milk from the age of 6 months to 2 years or more.

The importance of sound infant feeding based on locally available and affordable foods is clearly indicated in relation to the high rate of malnutrition in many countries, with deaths resulting directly or from added infections. In addition, the delayed damage of malnutrition (p.65) also calls for this aspect of maternal and child health programmes to receive top priority.

8
Protein–energy malnutrition

Michael Gurney, Derrick B. Jelliffe and Erasmus Harland

Growth in young children in the tropics

Many tropical children of poorer groups, living under both village and town conditions, show the following quite abnormal growth, as judged by their weight in the early years of life.

First 6 months of life

Breast-fed babies usually grow excellently for the first 4 to 6 months of life. Sufficient protein, energy (measured in calories or joules) and vitamins is supplied by a good flow of clean breast milk, together with the baby's body stores (obtained during fetal life); also the child is protected from many infections by antibodies obtained from the mother during pregnancy (p.6) and by cells and protective substances in breast milk (p.54).

Protein–energy malnutrition (PEM) is never found in a young baby who is satisfactorily breast-fed. If dilute gruels are given in the first month or two of life, breast-feeding will fall off rapidly, and one type of severe PEM — marasmus — may well result, often in the first 6 months (or earlier). This pattern is common in impoverished urban environments.

Second 6 months of life

After 4 to 6 months of age, breast milk alone is no longer sufficient for the child's needs. The first added food is usually a porridge. If the porridge is dilute, it does not provide enough energy; if it is not given with animal products, legumes or vegetables, it will be too low in iron, vitamins and protein; and if it is not very carefully prepared, it will carry organisms that can result in diarrhoea. Growth often starts to falter at this age.

Second and third years of life

This period is often marked by long periods with poor growth, or even no growth, or loss of weight. This is due to the low quality diet (e.g. small quantities of breast milk, limited amounts of nutritious foods, such as cow's milk, meat, fish or legumes such as beans), and to the numerous infections that may occur (e.g. measles, diarrhoea, malaria, chest infection, intestinal worms.).

Severe protein–energy malnutrition (PEM)

Severe protein–energy malnutrition comprises a range of conditions. One severe form of PEM is kwashiorkor (the child is somewhat underweight and always has oedema). The other type of severe PEM is marasmus (severe underweight below 60 per cent of the reference weight for age, but with no oedema). Intermediate severe conditions occur.

Many children have mild or moderate malnutrition in which they adapt to their inadequate diet by growing slowly and often being somewhat lethargic. These children are particularly susceptible to such infectious diseases as diarrhoea and may go on to develop the more severe forms of PEM.

Kwashiorkor

Definition

Kwashiorkor is a form of severe PEM, most usually occurring in early childhood, usually between the ages of 1 and 3 years. It is characterized by oedema and growth failure.

Causation

The main cause seems to be a diet that is very low in protein (especially in animal protein), consisting mainly of bulky, staple foods (p.61), mainly supplying some calories.

Reasons for a poor diet

A poor diet may have been given by the mother for one or more reasons: (i) poverty; (ii) lack of knowledge that children need a high-protein and energy diet during this period of rapid growth; (iii) cultural attitudes about certain foods (e.g. unwillingness to give milk, eggs, fish, meat or legumes (beans) to young children for a variety of incorrect reasons, such as because they are thought to produce worms), or an overemphasis on certain 'cultural super-foods', e.g. rice in South-East Asia, and banana in parts of Uganda.

Infections

Various infections may also assist in producing kwashiorkor, such as diarrhoea, which prevents absorption of food (p.102), intestinal worms (p.110), and respiratory infections, including tuberculosis (p.165) and whooping cough (p.135), which increase the body's need for energy and nutrients, and may affect appetite.

Special causes

Other situations that may be partly responsible for a poorly fed child developing kwashiorkor are: (i) lack of breast milk, as can occur if the mother dies or is seriously ill, if the child is 'displaced' from the breast by another pregnancy, if breast milk (and other food) has to be 'shared', as with twins, or if the mother leaves the child at home while she goes out to work and does not breast-feed; and (ii) abrupt stopping of breast-feeding, both in the home and especially if it is the custom to send the child away to stay with grandparents (with resulting misery and poor appetite).

Disease picture

The clinical signs of kwashiorkor vary somewhat from child to child and also in different parts of the world, but can be divided into those (1) always present, (2) usually present, and (3) occasionally present.

1. *Always present.* The following signs are always present and are all that is needed to make a diagnosis in a 1–3-year-old child who has probably been having a largely carbohydrate diet.

(a) *Oedema.* Swelling of the feet and lower legs due to oedema. Often also of the hands, lower back and, occasionally, the face. This is the most important diagnostic feature of true kwashiorkor.

(b) *Growth failure.* As shown by a low body weight even if oedema is present.

(c) *Wasted muscles but subcutaneous fat retained.* The child uses up his muscles to provide protein, and because of biochemical changes, his fat cannot be used for energy or growth.

(d) *Misery.* Difficult to measure but shown at first by peevishness and a whining cry, later by lack of interest.

2. *Usually present.* One or more of the following signs are usually present, but none is absolutely necessary to make a diagnosis.

(a) *Hair changes.* Lightness of colour (brown, reddish, nearly white, etc.); straightness; sparseness; silkiness; easily pulled out.

(b) *Light-coloured skin.* The whole body, or more often the face may be lighter in colour than in a healthy child.

(c) *Loose stools.* This may occur from failure of digestion of food, especially sugars.

(d) *Moderate anaemia.* If anaemia is severe, it usually suggests an associated infection with hookworm or malaria.

3. *Occasionally present.* One or more of the following signs are occasionally present, but none is absolutely needed to make a diagnosis.

(a) *'Flaky-paint' rash.* Dark-coloured patches of skin, which flake off leaving very light-coloured skin or even ulcers beneath. This can occur almost anywhere on the body, but is often seen on the backs of legs and buttocks.

(b) *Ulcers and cracks.* Small skin ulcers are often present, especially over pressure points. These may be deep cracks in the skin, especially behind and around the ears.

(c) *Signs of associated vitamin deficiency*, e.g. sore angles of the mouth and a bright-red tongue from lack of riboflavin.

(d) *Large liver.* The edge of the liver may be an inch (some 2.5 cm) below the rib margin. The enlargement is due to fatty change.

Differential diagnosis

This is usually not difficult, as kwashiorkor is much the commonest cause of oedema in the 1–3-year age group in most tropical countries.

1. *Hookworm disease* (p.110). Oedema is present, together with severe anaemia (sometimes with heart failure) and with the stools full of hookworm ova. The test for occult blood in the stools is usually positive. The skin shows generalized pallor, but is otherwise normal. (Diagnosis may be difficult in some cases when both conditions are present at the same time.)

2. *Nephrosis* is a kidney disease showing severe oedema, but with no signs of kwashiorkor and with the urine full of albumin. Ascites may be present in nephrosis, but does not usually occur in kwashiorkor.

Nutritional marasmus

Definition

Nutritional marasmus is a form of severe protein–energy malnutrition, usually occurring in the first 3 years of life. It is different from kwashiorkor. Two forms of marasmus occur:

early (usually in the first year of life) and late (occurring from 1–3 years or older).

Causation

The main cause is starvation, due to a diet severely lacking both in protein and in calories. The most common reasons for starvation are as follows.

1. *Inadequate bottle-feeding*. This can occur if the mother dies or abandons her child. Often the mother starts unnecessary bottle-feeding because she believes incorrectly that her own milk is 'inadequate' or 'too thin' (p.58). The mother may not be able to afford adequate milk or formula, so that she prepares over-dilute feeds. Also, if the feeding utensils, especially bottles, are dirty, the baby may get infective diarrhoea, which contributes to the development of marasmus. Inadequate bottle-feeding is the commonest cause of early marasmus.

2. *Starvation as treatment*. Sometimes nutritional marasmus may be produced by too long a period of starvation of children with infective diarrhoea. Children should have their diet restricted for as short a time as possible, usually not longer than 12 hours.

3. *Failure to introduce mixed diet*. 'Late' marasmus can occur in children receiving prolonged breast-feeding alone. In some parts of the world, 'late marasmus' is common, due to cultural delays in introducing other foods, and poverty, with rising food prices with inflation. After 4–6 months, other foods are needed in addition to breast-milk (p.61).

Disease picture

1. *Always present*. (i) Growth failure as shown by body weight, which is extremely low for age or height; (ii) wasting of both muscles and subcutaneous fat, as the diet has been low in calories as well as protein. In severe cases, the face has a 'little old man' appearance.

2. *Sometimes present*. (i) Loose stools, often because of infective diarrhoea; (ii) hair changes similar to those of kwashiorkor can occur but are much less marked, and very light-coloured hair is unusual; (iii) signs of associated vitamin deficiency; (iv) dehydration from infective diarrhoea.

Comparison with kwashiorkor

In contrast to kwashiorkor, children with nutritional marasmus: (i) are often under 1 year old; (ii) are obviously thin and wasted; (iii) have no oedema; (iv) are not miserable; and (v) have a good appetite.

Children whose weights are less than 60 per cent of reference weight for age who have oedema are diagnosed as having marasmic kwashiorkor and form an intermediate group.

Treatment of severe protein–energy malnutrition

Even though marasmus and kwashiorkor have very different clinical signs, the treatment is the same for each and for marasmic kwashiorkor.

Children with kwashiorkor are in danger of sudden death and thus need the best possible care and supervision. Children with marasmus often show very slow progress, with treatment sometimes taking weeks before satisfactory growth starts. The diarrhoea or other infections that often accompany severe PEM may be life threatening.

There are four main principles of treatment in all cases, but the way in which they can be carried out will vary with the severity of the case and with local medical resources, especially whether there are good hospital facilities.

1. Supply a high-energy diet with all the nutrients (especially protein) in proportion in a digestible, easily given (usually liquid) form.

2. Treat infections — respiratory, skin, malaria, hookworm, etc. — as soon as considered safe to do so.

3. Treat diarrhoea (and its associated mineral deficiencies) by emergency rehydration, if necessary (preferably using the oral route, p.106). This may mean a short delay before the high-energy–high nutrient diet can be started.

4. Ensure love, attention and affectionate contact ('TLC') with mothers (if present) or others, including the health staff.

The first week of treatment

The first few days of treatment are concentrated on medical management. Dehydration and mineral imbalance must be corrected first (p.106). In a severe case, the child's heart and kidneys may not be functioning well; the usual signs of an infection may not show themselves; both his blood sugar and his body temperature may drop very low, so he must be kept warm. Dilute feeds that do not provoke vomiting or diarrhoea should be given. Half-strength milk formula is very suitable. The feeds should be given little but often (around 12 times a day, every 2 hours). This could put a great strain on medical staff unless the mother or other relative is involved in management of the sick child. Breast-feeding should not be stopped. If the child will not eat, a nasogastric tube may be used for feeding.

As soon as possible, as the child's appetite improves, the strength of the formula should be increased (to full-strength milk mixture, for example, within 2 or 3 days). At the latest, before the end of the first week of treatment if the oedema has resolved, the child should be taking a high-energy milk mixture. The number of feeds can be reduced.

For the first 4 to 5 days of treatment, 125 ml of feed should be given per kg body weight per day (approximately 2 fl oz/lb). For example, a 4.5 kg (10 lb) child would need 4.5 × 125 = 560 ml/kg (10 × 2 = 20 fl oz/lb) of feed in one day. After this period, the quantity of feed should be increased to 150 ml/kg per day. This can be given as six feeds (i.e. 25 ml/kg per feed every 4 hours).

High-energy milk mixtures

Full-strength milk mixtures can be made from any milk mixed with oil, sugar and water. Table 8.1 sets out the quantities

Table 8.1 How to prepare full-strength milk feeds

Types of milk	Milk		Oil		Sugar		Water
	g	ml	g	ml	g	ml	(boiled/cooled)
Cow's/goat's milk	-	500	25	30	65	75	
Buffalo's/sheep's milk	-	450	15	20	50	55	
Skimmed milk powder	50	100	40	45	65	75	Make up to
Full-cream milk powder	70	150	25	30	60	65	1000 ml
Evaporated milk	205	190	25	30	60	65	
K-Mix 2*	75	80	50	55	15	20	
Yoghurt*	-	500	30	35	65	75	

* K-Mix 2 (calcium caseinate–skimmed milk powder–cane sugar) is distributed by UNICEF for treatment of PEM. Either K-mix 2 or yoghurt can be used if the child is thought to be unable to digest milk sugar (lactose) because of the diminished production of lactase (the intestinal secretion that digests lactose), because of the PEM itself, and/or because of associated intestinal infections.

required both by weight (in grams) and by volume (in millilitres). To make a half-strength formula, simply dilute the full-strength formula with a further 1000 ml of cool boiled water.

These formulae are ideally prepared in an electric blender. However, an egg-whisk or fork, will do; in this case, if powdered milk is being used, the milk, sugar and oil should be mixed to a smooth paste, the boiled and cooled water should be added to this paste little by little, and mixed in with the egg-beater or fork.

Method of feeding

Depending upon appetite and co-operation, the child may be fed by cup, spoon or by intragastric tube (at least for the first few days). The last-mentioned is very valuable in some cases as, with careful handling, it is safe, gets around the problem of the child's poor appetite and lack of interest, and is a great saving of nursing time.*

Minerals

Body potassium and magnesium are often low in children with kwashiorkor because of loss in loose stools, and because they are needed for the rebuilding of muscle during recovery. When available mineral mixture should be given three times daily, mixed with the feeds, to all cases of kwashiorkor admitted to the the ward. Each dose should consist of 0.5 g of potassium chloride and 0.1 g magnesium hydroxide. Sometimes, this mixture is added to the milk feeds.

Iron

Children with PEM, especially kwashiorkor, are often very anaemic (often partly due to malaria, hookworm or sickle cell

---

Tube feeding. Plastic tubing (size 2, internal diameter 1 mm) can be employed for intragastric feeds for severe cases of protein–energy malnutrition.

The required length of tubing (usually 45–60 cm; 18–24 inches) can be roughly estimated by measuring the distance from the front of the child's hair in the midline to the lower end of the sternum and doubling it. It is not necessary to sterilize new tubing before the first feed. The end of the tube should be smoothed by rubbing on sandpaper or by applying the flame of a match for a second.

The tube is lubricated with water and passed through a nostril into the stomach. The tubing can be fixed across the cheek in the direction of the ear with pieces of strapping. It can be left in place for several days, or even up to a week, because it is narrow and does not cause irritation.

Syringe. Three-hourly feeds can be given slowly by a syringe through an injection needle which fits the tube (size 18 BWC). Initially, and before each feed, the tube should be tested with a little boiled water. The child's arms should be splinted to prevent removal of the tube.

Some plastic tubing becomes soft when boiled. It must be removed carefully from the hot water as pressure may cause flattening. Tubing that can be boiled repeatedly is to be preferred.

anaemia). In all cases, iron and folic acid supplementation is desirable, after they have recovered from the acute phase.

Associated conditions

Infection
1. Children with severe protein–energy malnutrition with skin ulceration or infection, and/or symptoms or signs of respiratory infections, and all very severe cases, should be given antibiotics straight away.

2. In highly malarious areas, a 3-day course of chloroquine by mouth is given. If the child is vomiting or is unconscious, then the first dose of chloroquine is given intramuscularly (p.120).

3. Intestinal worms should be treated when the child begins to recover and is eating well (p.110).

4. Other infections should be treated as indicated (e.g. tuberculosis). Tuberculosis may be difficult to diagnose (p.135) but may have been treated on suspicion. *After recovery*, the use of the tuberculin test will show whether the suspicion was right or not, and treatment should be continued or stopped, as appropriate.

Vitamin A   In parts of the world where vitamin A deficiency (p.96) is common, it may show itself as a child starts to recover from PEM. Children in such areas should be given prophylactic doses of vitamin A (p.98) orally or by intramuscular injection of a water-soluble preparation.

Later treatment

Recovery should commence within a week. In kwashiorkor, this is shown by oedema beginning to disappear, the child taking interest in his surroundings, weight gain (following an initial loss, if there was oedema).

At this time, mainly medical management gives way to dietary therapy and preparation for the return home.

1. The diet should be very high in energy and other nutrients, including protein, vitamins and minerals.

2. As soon as possible, the diet should use foods readily available to the family (but maintaining the high-energy input), based on the principle of multimixes (p.61).

3. Key family members should be educated in the diet to be followed on return home (p.61) and in the prevention of infections (pp.190, 201).

4. Co-operation and assistance of local authorities, such as the Social Welfare Officer or Chief etc., should be sought where there has been a family breakdown.

The formula used in the initial treatment can now be increased in nutrient density to the levels shown in Table 8.2.

The child should receive 160 ml of the high-energy milk feed (containing over 200 calories per 100 g) per kg (2.5 fl oz/lb) body weight per day. He should be fed 4-hourly, day and night at first. With such a schedule he will put on weight extremely fast. This means he can get home quickly and is at low risk of acquiring infections.

After 2 weeks of treatment, or earlier if necessary, local family foods can be progressively introduced into the child's diet while maintaining a high-energy feed.

Table 8.2 How to prepare high-energy milk feeds

Types of milk	Milk		Oil		Sugar		Water
	g	ml	g	ml	g	ml	(boiled/cooled)
Cow's/goat's milk	900	900	55	60	70	80	
Buffalo's/sheep's milk	800	800	30	35	65	75	
Skimmed milk powder	90	180	85	95	65	75	Make up to
Full-cream milk powder	120	270	55	60	65	75	1000 ml
Evaporated milk	450	430	50	55	70	80	
K-Mix 2	120	130	85	95	35	40	
Yoghurt	900	900	65	70	70	80	

Rehabilitation

Severely affected children, including those with extreme oedema, severe muscle wasting, marked misery, and skin signs, should be treated as emergencies and admitted with their mothers to a reasonably equipped and staffed hospital. However, if good hospital accommodation is not available, such children can be treated in nutrition rehabilitation centres (p.220), or in their homes, under the supervision of primary health care workers (p.215), using home-prepared multimixes (p.61).

Severely malnourished children are always wasted; that is to say, they have a low body weight compared with their height. With successful treatment, they put on weight very fast, but grow taller only slowly. Intensive management based on the high-energy diet and treatment of infections should continue until the child achieves the normal weight for his height.

Once the child is about the normal weight for height (Table 8.3), high-energy feeding is no longer needed. In fact, his appetite will probably fall off when he reaches this level. This is where informed care by the mother, supported by a good primary health care service (p.215), is so important, if relapse is to be prevented.

In many parts of the world, many families eat only twice a day. The mother should then be especially instructed to feed her child four times daily. An underweight child needs snacks as well.

Mothers should not usually be advised to make milk powder into liquid milk, owing to the danger of causing diarrhoea from infection and wrong preparation. Dried skimmed milk is especially dangerous in this respect and, if used, must be reconstituted with vegetable oil.

When the child is thought well enough (or immediately in very mild cases), precise advice must be given on improving and widening the child's diet on local foods obtainable by the mother — including animal products, such as fresh and dried milk, fish, eggs and meat, and vegetable foods, often as

Table 8.3 Average normal weights for heights of infants and children (both sexes)

Height (cm)	Equivalent weight (kg), average	Height (cm)	Equivalent weight (kg), average
49	3.2	86	11.9
50	3.3	87	12.1
51	3.5	88	12.3
52	3.7	89	12.6
53	3.9	90	12.8
54	4.1	91	13.0
55	4.3	92	13.2
56	4.5	93	13.5
57	4.8	94	13.7
58	5.0	95	13.9
59	5.3	96	14.2
60	5.6	97	14.5
61	5.8	98	14.7
62	6.1	99	15.0
63	6.4	100	15.3
64	6.7	101	15.6
65	7.0	102	16.0
66	7.3	103	16.3
67	7.6		
68	7.9		
69	8.2		
70	8.4		
71	8.7		
72	9.0		
73	9.2		
74	9.5		
75	9.7		
76	9.9		
77	10.1		
78	10.3		
79	10.5		
80	10.7		
81	10.9		
82	11.1		
83	11.3		
84	11.5		
85	11.7		

Note: these figures are only approximate as individual children vary in body height.

mixtures, especially beans, and other legumes, cereals and dark green leafy vegetables. Oil and sugar ('compact calories') are very important for underweight children (p.61).

Prevention of protein–energy malnutrition

Long term

This will be concerned with such wide activities as the following.

1. Improving the country's food supply to ensure that an adequate and balanced supply is available when and where it is needed ('food availability').

2. Improving the economic level of the country, and the money available for people to buy foods, or land on which to grow them, ('food affordability').

3. Improving the general level of education so that parents, especially mothers, understand the importance of the correct feeding of their children.

4. Primary health care, including maternal and child welfare services (p.215) for nutrition and health supervision and treatment, for education and for the prevention of infectious disease (i.e. by immunization, p.201). This, in turn, is related to the need to educate health staff in paediatrics, especially nutrition.

Education

This involves teaching all sections of the community, especially fathers and mothers, to make the best use of the foods available (including breast-feeding), to make use of available primary health care services, and to grow local foods in their own gardens.

Supply of special infant food

Such processed foods are expensive to provide, but they can be useful. They should be mixed with local dishes, especially soft pastes or 'multimixes'. They should not replace breast milk. Special categories, such as twins, may have to be given particular attention.

Practical plan of infant feeding

There are five rules which, if kept, can largely prevent protein–energy malnutrition.

1. *Breast-feed at least until 1–2 years* (p.66). Breast-feeding prolonged into the second year of life is the traditional and historical way of feeding human babies. The milk of even poorly-fed tropical mothers in late breast-feeding is relatively normal in nutrient content, although somewhat decreased in quantity. For poorer mothers (among whose children kwashiorkor occurs) prolonged breast-feeding is to be encouraged (up to 1 or 2 years, depending upon the local customary pattern — providing another pregnancy does not occur and the mother is otherwise medically fit). The breast milk will supply a small, but valuable, extra amount of nutrients to the child. In addition, detailed advice must be given to the mother in order to improve her own diet while pregnant and during the period of prolonged breast-feeding, especially with local dishes prepared from a mixture of foods including beans and dark green leafy vegetables.

2. *Start porridge at 4 months.* Breast milk alone is completely adequate up to and beyond this time. If the infant fails to gain weight normally before this time, the cause should be looked for — it should not be assumed that the breast-milk is inadequate. Porridge, paste or gruels should be as thick as possible.

3. *Provide a three-plank bridge.* The idea has been found useful that a 'nutrient bridge' — of soft semisolid or solid foods — has to be made to carry the children over the dangerous period between 4–9 months and 2–3 years. The

three planks are as follows.

(a) *Continued breast-feeding*

(b) *Use all available animal food sources.* Although usually foods of animal origin are both expensive and in short supply, efforts must be made to encourage mothers to use all available supplies, including fresh or dried milk, fish, eggs and meat. The more digestible of these should be introduced first. Various food attitudes and prejudices (p.12) may have to be overcome. It is probable that, in many cases, there will not be much food of animal origin for the child. However, even very small extra amounts are of importance.

(c) *Use vegetable mixtures.* While the first semisolid food given (all over the world) is usually a gruel or paste prepared from the staple, this should soon be followed by a gruel or paste made of a mixture of locally available vegetable foods. This mixture will normally be based on a cereal (e.g. millet, maize, rice, etc) and a legume (e.g. beans or peas). Together, these two types of food supply all the ingredients (essential amino acids) of animal protein. How these mixtures are to be prepared, suitable recipes, and the proportions to be used, will have to be worked out locally, depending on available foods, cooking methods, customs, etc. Often one can start with a 3 : 1 mixture (cereal or other staple to legume) and gradually increase to 2 : 1. The value of these mixtures is improved greatly by the addition of even small amounts of dried or fresh milk or other animal products. Such 'triple mixes' are composed of staple, legume, and animal product, and ideally should also include dark green leafy vegetables and a source of 'compact calories' (such as oil or fat).

4. *Give children four good meals a day.* Their stomachs are small, but their need for food is great, especially for calories.

5. *Feed sick children.* Sick children need extra nutrients and energy to repair body tissues. However, they often have a low appetite that may be aggravated by a sore mouth (as in measles or thrush). There may also be taboos against certain

foods during illness, or a belief that they should be starved or put on a very limited diet. Sick children should, in fact, be coaxed to eat good quality food. When they are better, they will need extra food. They are not completely recovered until they have regained the weight lost when they were ill.

9
Anaemia

Charlotte Neumann

Anaemia is a condition in which there is a decreased amount of haemoglobin in the body. This substance is carried inside red blood cells, so that anaemia will occur if each of the red cells contains too little haemoglobin or if the number of red cells is low. Anaemia is among the top ten causes of death in childhood. It is one of the most common conditions affecting children not only in the tropics, but in temperate zones. There are many causes of anaemia and often more than one cause is present at one time.

The normal full-term baby is born with a high haemoglobin of about 18–20 g per 100 ml [decilitre (dl)], which was necessary for the fetus while in utero. However, after birth, this level of haemoglobin is no longer necessary, and a large number of red cells are destroyed so that the haemoglobin level falls to about 11 g/dl by the time the child is 4 months old. From that age onward, the level slowly rises and, when the child is 7 years old, it will have reached 13–14 g/dl (Table 9.1).

During the early days of life, when red cells are being destroyed, the iron they contain is stored in the liver and bone marrow to be used to make haemoglobin later on. As the child grows, the amount of blood in the body increases so that more cells and haemoglobin have to be made; thus a baby at 1 year of age may have 3 times the amount of blood it had when it was born. The body makes haemoglobin from iron, protein and other important nutrients obtained from the child's food and body stores.

Why anaemia causes problems

Oxygen is carried to the tissues by haemoglobin in the red blood cells, and carbon dioxide is carried away. In severe

83

Table 9.1 Normal mean and lower limits: haematological values in children

	Haemoglobin (g/dl)*		Haematocrit (%)	
	Mean	Lower limit (-2 S.D.)	Mean	Lower limit (-2 S.D.)
Newborn	16.8	13.5	55	45
1 week to 6 months	13.0	11.0	36	31
6 months to 2 years	12.5	11.0	37	33
2–4 years	12.5	11.0	38	34
4–8 years	13.0	11.5	39	35
8–11 years	13.5	12.0	40	36
11–14 years: female	13.5	12.0	41	36
male	14.0	12.5	43	37
14–18 years: female	14.0	12.0	41	36
male	16.0	14.0	46	38

* Add 0.2 g/dl of haemoglobin for each 750 m (2500 ft) above sea level.

anaemia, tissues may not receive enough oxygen. Muscle performance and work capacity are decreased in anaemia. In young children, especially with iron deficiency, the nervous system may be affected. They do not learn as well as non-anaemic children as they are not able to concentrate. Infections are more common and the body defences against infection may be decreased. The heart has to work harder to pump an increased volume of blood and oxygen to the body. With severe anaemia, heart failure can occur.

Diagnosis of anaemia

The diagnosis of anaemia varies in the different age groups, as does the relative importance of different causes. Children between 1 and 3 years old and pregnant women are at the greatest risk. If the common causes of anaemia can be determined, the treatment can be started with some assurance that it is likely to be effective, even if special laboratory results are not available. Primary health care workers can be trained to recognize and treat anaemia effectively. Patients

who do not respond can then be referred for further
investigation and treatment.

History

It is important to identify certain risk factors that may make a
child susceptible to anaemia, for example, twins, prematurity
and bleeding from the cord.

In later infancy and in the toddler age group, when and
which solids were added to the diet; particularly eggs, cereal,
soups, meat, dark green leafy vegetables? What is the
approximate frequency (e.g. times per week these are eaten)?

In terms of infections or infestations, does the child have
grossly bloody stools, frequent diarrhoea or obvious
parasites? Has the child received any malaria prophylaxis or
had known bouts of malaria? Is hookworm a problem in the
community? Is there any obvious familial history of severe
anaemia in any of the siblings or parents?

Clinical signs and symptoms

While some anaemias may give rise to special signs, such as
painful swollen fingers in sickle-cell anaemia, all show the
following general signs:

Slowly developing anaemia

Paleness (which can be judged best from the appearance of
the lips, finger-nails and toe-nails, the palms of the hands, the
tongue and the conjunctiva), a rapid heart rate, lack of
energy, poor appetite and listlessness are generally present.

Rapidly developing anaemia

Paleness, which is often very marked, a very rapid heart rate
and a weak, soft pulse, rapid respiration, cyanosis and
cardiac failure with oedema and enlarged liver are present.

With haemolysis, one sees a yellow hue or jaundice, best detected in the skin and conjunctiva.

Laboratory diagnosis

For screening purposes, the simplest measurements are either the haemoglobin or haematocrit (see Table 9.1). In addition, a blood smear can help to diagnose the type of anaemia, and a sickle-cell test is needed to diagnose sickle-cell anaemia. Stool examination can reveal the presence of hookworm ova (p.110).

Classification of anaemia

Anaemia may be due to one or more factors, particularly in very poor living circumstances. The major causes are outlined in Table 9.2. The majority of anaemias are due to decreased blood production, increased blood destruction, or blood loss. The more common types of anaemia are described below.

Table 9.2 Classification of anaemia in childhood: common causes

A. *Decreased red cell production*
    1. Depletion of building blocks — 'nutritional anaemias'
        Iron, folate, protein, B12, etc.
    2. Bone marrow failure
        Primary marrow aplasia or hypoplasia
        Secondary marrow aplasia due to toxins and chronic
        infection

B. *Blood loss*
    1. Acute haemorrhage — placental, cord, viscera, haemorrhagic
        disease of the newborn
    2. Chronic haemorrhage — hookworm, amoebiasis,
        gastrointestinal disease

C. *Excessive red cell destruction*
    1. Infection — malaria, sepsis, kala azar
    2. Hereditary — sickle-cell disease, thalassaemia, G6PD with
        sensitivity to drugs (sulphonamides, primaquine, fava beans
        etc.)

Newborn period

The presence of anaemia in the newborn period may often be due to life-threatening problems and needs to be recognised as a problem. The main types of anaemia in the newborn period are due to acute blood loss and to haemolytic destruction of red blood cells. Acute blood loss may occur prior to delivery or just after delivery and in the first few days of life. The infant may appear pale, with a rapid or weak pulse, blue (cyanotic) because of lack of oxygen and rapid respirations. Haemolysis of the infant's blood may occur rapidly with the above symptoms and signs, but in addition the infant will develop jaundice or yellow discoloration of the skin and conjunctiva.

In the newborn period, very early clamping of the cord may deprive the infant of over 100 ml of blood. Acute blood loss may occur from an improperly tied cord stump. The above situations, except for early clamping of the cord, may require immediate life-saving transfusions.

Acute blood loss may also occur following a very traumatic delivery in which haemorrhages occur into the brain or abdominal organs.

Haemorrhagic disease of the newborn may be a cause of acute or subacute blood loss. Some infants between the second and eighth day of life develop decreased or absent ability to clot their blood because of low blood prothrombin, an important clotting factor. The infant may lose blood from the umbilical cord stump, vomit up blood, pass black tarry stools due to altered blood in the intestine, and develop shock with weak and rapid pulse. Transfusion and vitamin K (1 mg) given intramuscularly are life saving. A routine newborn practice in Western countries is to give vitamin K routinely to all newborns. The benefits of this practice are debatable and some feel that only infants who have had difficult delivery or are premature should be given vitamin K prophylactically. Only the natural oil preparation and not the synthetic vitamin K product should be used, as the latter has caused jaundice in susceptible infants.

Haemolytic disease of the newborn (erythroblastosis

foetalis) starts in utero. This occurs when the mother's blood group differs from her infant's so that the mother produces antibodies against her infant's red blood cells. These antibodies pass from her blood into the baby's circulation and cause the breakdown (haemolysis) of the infant's red cells.

Another cause of haemolytic anaemia in the newborn period which must be dealt with promptly is due to sepsis. This is caused by bacteria whose toxins cause breakdown of red blood cells. If the mother is at term, or near term, has clinical infection with fever or has had ruptured membranes for over 48 hours, jaundice and signs of anaemia in a listless baby within 48 to 72 hours of birth should raise serious concern about the presence of sepsis, and prompt diagnosis and antibiotic treatment may be lifesaving. These infants should be referred for hospital care, if possible.

Decreased red blood cell production due to nutritional deficiency

Nutritional anaemias are due to insufficient production of haemoglobin and red cells due to lack of 'building blocks'. Anaemia may be due to lack of nutrients in the diet, abnormal losses or excessive requirements. The main nutrient deficiencies in anaemia are iron, folic acid, protein, vitamin B_{12}, copper and pyridoxine. This may be due to inadequate intake in the diet, abnormal losses through chronic diarrhoea, poor intestinal absorption, certain parasites and blood loss and destruction.

Iron deficiency anaemia

Iron deficiency anaemia is the most common cause of anaemia throughout the world, with small, pale, poorly filled cells compared to normal red blood cells. Insufficient iron intake is the leading cause. Milk is a poor source of iron, and infants are at particular risk when no iron-containing solids are added to their diet until the second year of life. Low birth weight is also a factor as the infant is born with a smaller blood volume, with less circulating haemoglobin and with poor iron stores, than the normal-weight newborn. With rapid growth, the blood compartment is rapidly expanded and there is insufficient iron to make sufficient haemoglobin.

Although present in small amounts, iron from breast milk is much better absorbed than that from other milks. Vegetable sources of iron may be poorly absorbed. The absorption from wheat and soya is better than from rice or other vegetable sources, but iron is best absorbed from meat sources. Children with iron deficiency are listless, have anorexia and are irritable. Recent evidence in infants and young children showed that diminished learning ability occurs with iron deficiency, even in the absence of anaemia.

Iron deficiency in the newborn and in early infancy, as mentioned above, may be due to haemorrhage and blood loss early in life or because of low birth weight. Later in infancy and in childhood, iron deficiency is due largely to poor nutritional intake of iron and/or chronic loss as with hookworm or other intestinal parasites.

Folate deficiency

Next in prevalence to iron deficiency anaemia is megaloblastic anaemia due to folate deficiency and this is a common cause of anaemia in many parts of the world. The red blood cells are large and the white blood cells have multilobed nuclei. Mothers deficient in folic acid in their diet produce folic-acid-deficient milk, which can result in young infants between 3 and 5 months with severe megaloblastic anaemia and even heart failure. Infants given goat's milk are also at risk of folate deficiency anaemia as this is a poor source of folic acid. Folic acid is deficient when a diet lacks meat, eggs, and milk products which most of the world cannot afford. Dark green leafy vegetables are fortunately an excellent source of folate, as are yams, sweet potatoes and other fruits. Folate is destroyed in prolonged cooking.

Haemolysis, with rapid blood cell destruction and

formation increases the body's need for folic acid. This occurs with frequent bouts of malaria, sickle-cell disease and other forms of haemolytic anaemia. The presence of infection and diarrhoea with malabsorption also lower folic acid levels and body stores.

B_{12} deficiency anaemia

The blood picture with B_{12} deficiency is similar to that of folic acid deficiency, with megaloblasts and multilobed nuclei. However, neurological impairment also occurs. This is seen only where a strict vegetarianism is practised and in infancy where breast-milk is devoid of vitamin B_{12}. Also, a diet of raw fish containing a special tapeworm can also cause B_{12} deficiency.

Vitamin E deficiency

This is rarely seen in breast-fed infants but can be seen in infants who are given substitutes for breast-milk where butter fat is substituted with vegetable oil. Haemolytic anaemia occurs in these infants. It is made worse when iron is also given.

Increased destruction of red blood cells

Red blood cells can be destroyed (haemolysed) prematurely or more readily due to several causes, including sickle-cell disease in children of African descent (see below), the effect of some poisons (such as lead) and from severe infections (such as malaria and septicaemia).

Sickle-cell anaemia and trait

Because they are common in African children sickle-cell problems are emphasized here.

In sickle-cell anaemia, the red cells contain an abnormal

form of haemoglobin called haemoglobin S. If a child inherits haemoglobin S from one parent and normal adult haemoglobin A from the other parent, the child has sickle-cell trait, or SA anaemia. These children have no symptoms, and show only a positive sickling cell test. If the child gets haemoglobin S from both parents, he develops sickle-cell *disease*, or SS. Haemoglobin S under certain conditions forms crystals within the cells and the cells are destroyed rapidly by haemolysis, and the haemoglobin level falls abruptly with the development of a moderate to severe anaemia. Sickle cells can also cause blockage of blood vessels, causing a variety of signs and symptoms.

The child with sickle-cell disease (SS) may be well until 6 months of age. Thereafter, repeated attacks of fever, jaundice, anaemia and enlargement of the liver and spleen ensue. Sometimes, an infant will develop warm, swollen, painful fingers, toes, hands and feet. This is called the 'hand–foot' syndrome. Also, in the second year of life and thereafter, there may be enlargement of the skull which is very characteristic of sickle-cell disease and other chronic anaemias. This is due to blood formation in the bone marrow of the skull to try to keep up with blood cell destruction.

A sickle-cell crisis is a temporary worsening of the condition which is characterized by severe pain in the extremities, secondary to blocked vessels, and liver and spleen enlargement. Infection, dehydration and fever can cause these crises. Also, children with sickle-cell disease are very prone to serious bone infection or osteomyelitis and bloodstream infection. Children with sickle-cell disease also require increased folic acid.

Malaria

Malaria parasites invade red blood cells and then multiply within the cell. As they multiply and break out of the cell into the bloodstream, red blood cells are destroyed. Repeated bouts of malaria starting in early infancy can cause prolonged, increasingly severe anaemia.

Glucose 6-phosphate dehydrogenase (G 6-PD) deficiency

This deficiency is common among certain populations. G6 PD is an enzyme found in normal cells. Deficiency on a genetic basis is widespread among certain groups in Africa, Asia, and the Mediterranean countries. Usually there is no problem clinically, even with deficiency, unless the individual comes in contact with certain drugs, chemicals or infection. Such drugs as the sulphonamides, antimalarials such as primaquine, aspirin and certain foods such as fava beans can cause rapid haemolysis with resultant jaundice and anaemia.

Thalassaemia

Thalassaemia, also known as Mediterranean anaemia or Cooley's anaemia, is an inherited anaemia due to production of abnormal haemoglobin. The minor form causes no problems, but thalassaemia major, a severe form of the disease, leads to severe anaemia and even death due to defective red blood production, haemolysis and anaemia. Thalassaemia has been seen in groups living around the Mediterranean basin as well as in Iran, China, South-east Asia, and north of the Sahara, in Africa and in India.

The major forms of the disease first appear in the first 3–6 months of life. There are repeated bouts of haemolysis and anaemia with a rapidly enlarging spleen, with death often occurring by the age of 1 year. A less severe form has its onset after 1 year, but the outcome is nonetheless fatal. The skull may become enlarged in appearance with frontal and parietal enlargement (bossing) because of the bone marrow proliferation. The increased red blood cell production is an attempt by the body to keep up with the rapid destruction of red cells.

Thalassaemia minor produces a moderate degree of anaemia, often between 6 and 9 g/dl, in children and adolescents, with mild jaundice and splenic enlargement. Many of these children survive to adult life.

Decreased red blood cell production due to bone marrow problems

Various conditions can lead to decreased production of red cells, such as toxic drugs (chloramphenicol etc.).

Prevention and therapeutic approaches to childhood anaemia

Prevention

The approach to prevention of anaemia has many aspects. Starting with pregnant women, measures to ensure adequate maternal nutrition in pregnancy (and during breast-feeding) and to prevent low birth weight can promote adequate iron stores in the mother and infant. At the time of delivery, late cord clamping (after cord pulsations cease) and care in ligating the cord to prevent haemorrhage are important.

In terms of nutritional anaemia, parents need to be instructed on the advisability of introduction of iron- and protein-containing solids as well as foods rich in folate and vitamin B_{12} by 4 to 6 months, in addition to breast milk.

Malaria prophylaxis in young children will protect against anaemia due to malaria (p.117). Control in areas of mosquitoes will aid in prevention of malaria. The prevention of hookworm infection is also important (p.110).

Approach to treatment

Awareness of the leading causes of anaemia among various age groups for a given community allows for presumptive diagnosis and treatment of anaemia. For example, in a known malarious area, an infant or toddler would be given a combination of an iron preparation, folic acid and anti-malarial treatment. If, following a therapeutic trial, the anaemia does not respond, then referral for more detailed investigations is needed. This has been called the 'package

Table 9.3 Treatment of anaemia in children

A. Nutritional anaemias

Iron deficiency	Ferrous sulphate liquid Elemental iron in each: Fer-in-sol (25 mg/ml) Ferrous sulphate elixir (8-10 mg/ml)	6 mg/kg elemental iron in 3 divided doses for one month longer than return of haemoglobin to normal level (2-3 months total).
	Imferon (iron dextran) intramuscular iron	Haemoglobin deficit % × body wt (kg × 0.6)
	Transfusion – packed cells for severe anaemia and heart failure	Volume of packed cells (ml) per lb. of body wt. = Haemoglobin level (e.g. if Hg is 2 g/dl give 2 ml per lb of body weight of packed cells)
Folate deficiency	Folic acid orally	5 mg p.o. day for 7 to 14 days
Vitamin E deficiency	Vitamin E orally for low birth weight and/or in preterm infants	75-100 IU/24 hours in divided doses.
Protein deficiency	Protein plus adequate calories, iron and folate diet	1 g/kg protein/day
Haemorrhagic disease newborn	Vitamin K_1	1–2 mg Vit. K i.m.

B. Infestations and infections: malaria (p.117), hookworm (p.110)

C. Hereditary anaemias

Sickle cell	No specific treatment Transfusion as needed Folic acid if haemolysis occurring Crises	Treat for iron deficiency if present 1 mg/day
	Treat infection Keep hydrated acetaminophen for pain codeine (avoid aspirin if G6-Pd present)	Ampicillin and penicillin oral and IV fluids 60 mg/yr 3 mg/kg in divided doses for 24 hours
Thalassaemia	Transfusion to maintain Hg 8 to g/dl	10–15 ml/kg of packed cells

approach' and is suited for health centres or peripheral health services which rely on simple diagnostic measures. An outline of treatment is presented in Table 9.3.

Continuous follow-up is desirable for children under treatment for anaemia. It is important to see if treatment is or was effective so that 'failures' can be referred for further evaluation and treatment. Because of the rapid growth of young children, with rapid increase in the blood volume, periodic testing for anaemia is also important. The haemoglobin can often serve as a measure of nutritional level, as well as of height and weight (p78).

Key preventive measures in childhood anaemia involve nutrition education, improvement of sanitation, particularly for excreta disposal, malarial prophylaxis in young children, and control of mosquitoes. Community approaches to combatting childhood anaemia have also included fortification of foods, particularly with iron, with some promising results. However, the cost and difficulties of selecting a food widely used by young children usually make this impossible.

10
Vitamin A deficiency (xerophthalmia)

Susan Pettiss

Xerophthalmia is an eye disease caused by lack of vitamin A and by malnutrition. It most often strikes the under-6 age group in tropical countries where the customary diet consists only of rice, white maize, cassava, or other vitamin-deficient staples — children who do not get enough food and not the right kind of food. Children in poor families in the rural areas or the city slums are most affected. Often these children are not in easy reach of medical care and suffer from repeated infectious diseases and diarrhoea.

Definition

'Xerophthalmia' means 'dry eye disease', and is so called because of the appearance of the conjunctiva and cornea. A recent world review showed xerophthalmia to be very common in the Asian countries of Indonesia, India, Philippines and Bangladesh. The condition also occurs commonly in some regions of Africa, Latin America and the Caribbean.

Cause

The disease is caused by a deficiency of vitamin A which may result from:

(a) insufficiency of vitamin A in the diet (quality of the food);
(b) inadequacy of amount of food (quantity of food);
(c) inability of the body to use vitamin A;
(d) depletion of vitamin A from liver stores.

Vitamin A can be obtained from two sources. Certain foods, such as eggs, whole milk, liver and fish, provide the

96

vitamin directly to the body. Other foods, such as green leafy vegetables, carrots, tomatoes, mangoes and papaya, contain a substance (beta-carotene) which can be changed into vitamin A in the body and then absorbed. As long as a baby is fed with mother's milk, there is little danger of xerophthalmia. Often, however, when the baby is weaned, only rice or gruel is fed, so that the nutrients the baby needs are lacking.

Xerophthalmia is likely to occur in malnourished children, and often accompanies protein–energy malnutrition (PEM). There is also an important relationship between childhood infections and vitamin A deficiency. When a child becomes sick, he may lose his appetite and not get enough of the vitamin in the food eaten. Such illnesses often reduce the body's ability to absorb and use the vitamin in the food; with no intake, the vitamin stored in the liver becomes drained.

The diseases most associated with vitamin A deficiency are respiratory tract infections, childhood infectious diseases such as measles, roundworms, whooping cough, tuberculosis, and frequent and prolonged diarrhoea.

Disease picture

Often the first symptom of xerophthalmia is night blindness. Mothers are usually quick to recognize the problem as the child no longer moves about the house or village after dark, but sits in a corner, unable to find his food or toys. Recent research in Indonesia showed that, at least in that country, the mother's word could be relied upon as an accurate diagnosis when carefully questioned.

Bitot's spots on the conjunctiva are another early sign. These spots look like white, sticky foam on the white portion of the eye. They may vary in size, shape and location but almost always occur in both eyes.

As the disease progresses, the conjunctiva becomes dry and rough looking, a stage called 'conjunctival xerosis'. Corneal xerosis (dryness) may develop if the disease is not treated. The clear, transparent cornea covers the dark part of the eye, the iris and pupil. If it loses its transparency, it can result in partial or total blindness.

In more serious cases, the dryness may quickly give way to a softening of the cornea with bulging or rupture, and blindess. When corneal ulcers are still superficial, prompt treatment with a large dose of vitamin A may produce rapid healing with little or no loss of sight, but once they perforate, a white scar (leucoma) causes complete blindness. However, sometimes it is possible to save one eye by giving a vitamin A dose even though the other is lost.

Treatment

Early recognition of xerophthalmia is essential, as is the risk of young children developing the condition, especially in some areas. This is a medical emergency requiring immediate administration of large amounts of vitamin A, which can be given by mouth or by injection. It is important, however, that the vitamin A injected be waterbased (*not* the oily preparation). It has been found that 200 000 iu vitamin A given by mouth on two days successively is as effective as an injection, and much more practical. The treatment schedule recommended by WHO is as follows.

Children* with xerophthalmia or general illness or malnutrition

Immediately on diagnosis	200 000 iu vitamin A orally *or* 100 000 iu water-miscible vitamin A intramuscularly
Following day	200 000 iu vitamin A orally
Prior to discharge, or 1-2 weeks later	200 000 iu vitamin A orally

*For children less than 1 year of age reduce all doses by one-half.

Severely ill and malnourished children in communities where xerophthalmia is known to occur should be given the large dose of vitamin A whether or not they are showing signs of the disease. Where the vitamin A is not available, the child should be immediately given foods rich in the vitamin, such as dairy products, fish, liver oil, etc., and, if these are not accessible, dark green leafy vegetables and red, yellow and orange-coloured fruits or vegetables.

Proper attention should also be given to correcting protein-energy malnutrition or associated infections, if these are also present.

Recent research has shown a close relationship of measles with xerophthalmia, especially in Africa. Therefore, it is recommended that measles therapy should include additional dietary intake of vitamin A and high dose of vitamin A when available.

Prevention

The blind child in a developing country faces a most difficult life. These are usually children of the poorest families, in the poorest sections of the poorest countries. They live in countries which can least afford to give them the special services and education needed to enable blind persons to lead a full life. The large size of the problem is indicated by an estimate that more than a quarter of a million preschool Asian children lose their sight from xerophthalmia each year.

This is a tragedy, as *nutritional blindness is preventable*. It does not exist in many parts of the world and it could become a thing of the past everywhere.

Long-range prevention

The obvious solution to the problem of nutritional blindness is the improvement of the socio-economic conditions so that increased standards of living will enable all families to have sufficient caloric and nutritious diets. In the meantime, however, there are some steps that can be taken to make the best use of existing foods. In most countries, there *are* vegetables and fruit which are available at little or no cost and found in sufficient quantity. If the amount of dark green leafy vegetables and suitable fresh fruits eaten by vulnerable children could be increased, there is reason to believe the problem would be greatly improved.

Short-term prevention

In order to prevent vitamin A deficiency in children in the present circumstances, immediate short-term measures must be undertaken in some countries where the problem is very common. Long-range plans must go on at the same time. Immediate preventive measures include distribution of high-dosage (200 000 iu) vitamin A in liquid or capsule form (capsules are often made available by UNICEF) to preschool-age populations known to be at high risk. Parts of the following preventive programme can be used in high-risk areas.

Infants — 6 months of age. If the infant is not breast-fed or if at risk because the mother did not receive vitamin A at delivery or during the following 4 weeks, 100 000 iu vitamin A may be given at any one time during the first 6 months.

All other children under 6 years of age. 200 000 iu vitamin A orally every 4–6 months.

Pregnant women. Large doses of vitamin A should *not* be given at any time during pregnancy. (During the first 3 months there is strong evidence that congenital abnormalities may result. In the last 6 months there is the possibility of excessive transfer of vitamin A to the fetus.) Women considered to be vitamin A deficient may safely be given small frequent doses throughout pregnancy and lactation, not to exceed 10 000 iu daily.

Women at and after birth of child. 200 000 iu vitamin A should be given by mouth to mothers immediately after the birth of the child or during the 4 weeks following delivery. (A single dose has been shown to raise the vitamin A level in breast milk significantly for at least 1 month.)

Lactating women. Large doses of vitamin A should *not* be administered during lactation. (A further conception may take place at any time during lactation, and a large dose of vitamin A may damage the fetus.)

Xerophthalmia has complicated causes, and is usually associated with complicating childhood infection and/or general malnutrition. Improvement in public health programmes is essential to assist in reducing infections and malnutrition (including measles vaccination, where feasible), to supply vitamin A and health education, and to detect and treat cases early, through primary health care services.

A combination of nutrition and health education is always needed, with preventive distribution of vitamin A for young children in areas where xerophthalmia is very common. Training of medical, nutrition and child welfare staff to recognize the disease, to treat it and to help mothers know how to prevent it is essential.*

*Slide sets suitable for training different types of staff are available from the Helen Keller International Inc., 15 West Sixteenth Street, New York, NY 10011, USA.

11

Diarrhoeal disease in early childhood

Robert Cook

Importance of diarrhoea

In almost all developing countries diarrhoea is a very common illness of infants and young children. In many countries, it is the main cause of death in this age group. Children die mainly of dehydration in acute diarrhoea because they do not replace quickly enough the water and electrolytes (sodium, potassium etc.) lost in the stools and in vomiting, and therefore they go into a state of shock and coma and they die. Diarrhoea also kills infants directly, because repeated attacks are a major cause of PEM (protein-energy malnutrition), especially of the marasmic kind, and this also is a common problem in early childhood in many countries. Thus diarrhoea accounts directly and indirectly for between a quarter and a half of all sickness and deaths under the age of 5 years in the Third World. The peak age of incidence is from 6 months to 2 years in general, but where many babies under 6 months are bottle-fed, there can be many below that age also.

Definition of diarrhoea

As a rough guide, we can say that three or more *loose* or *watery* stools a day can be considered diarrhoea, but we cannot be too rigid about this. The mother's own knowledge of the child has to be taken into account as well, since she is the one who knows what the stools of the child are usually like.

The stools of breast-fed children are often softer and more frequent than those of bottle-fed children. This is *not* diarrhoea.

102

Causes of diarrhoea

The main cause of acute diarrhoea is infection of the intestines with viruses or bacteria. Much new knowledge about these micro-organisms has been acquired in the last decade or so. It seems that as well as the cholera *vibrio, Shigella, Salmonella* and enteropathogenic *Esch. coli*, other kinds of *Esch. coli* (enterotoxigenic) and also viruses, especially *rotavirus*, are very important. Less frequent as a cause are the protozoa, *Giardia* and *Entamoeba*. One worm, *Trichuris*, can also be a cause of diarrhoea.

In addition, acute diarrhoea sometimes occurs as a complication of measles, of malignant tertian malaria (p.117), and of other infections outside the gut such as tonsillitis, otitis media, and pneumonia. It is not known how often these other infections are truly due to the diseases in themselves, and how often they are due to simultaneous intestinal infection in a sick and weakened child, but in any case one should always look out for underlying conditions like these, and when they seem to be present, treat them appropriately.

Chronic diarrhoea is due sometimes to chronic infection of the gut, but more often to damage to the intestinal wall (epithelium) from a previous acute infection. Such damage to the epithelium can also occur as a result of kwashiorkor.

However, much of the problem occurs at the primary health care level in overcrowded urban clinics or isolated rural areas where stool examinations are not possible, especially for bacterial culture and determination of sensitivity to antibiotics. It is much more important to consider the cause of diarrhoea in the more fundamental sense, that it is due to the child swallowing viruses, bacteria, protozoa, eggs of worms etc. which come from somebody else's faeces. They get into the child's mouth from dirty hands, dirty food or milk, dirty water and dirty utensils, especially feeding bottles. Every health worker understands this, but he or she has to make sure that every mother knows it too. That would be a big step in preventing diarrhoea.

For avoiding diarrhoea in young babies under 6 months of age, it should be understood that the value of breast-feeding is not only in that it is free from harmful bacteria etc., but also it has many substances in it which specifically counterattack such micro-organisms as may nevertheless get into the gut (p.54).

The importance of dehydration and why it occurs

Treatment with antibiotics or with anti-diarrhoeal agents such as kaolin, pectin or opiates will have very little effect on the outcome of most cases of diarrhoea in young children. They will survive or die according to whether they avoid becoming dehydrated or not — that is, according to whether their water–electrolyte balance is maintained, or restored to normal if it is already affected. This is the most important point about the treatment of diarrhoeal disease.

The food and drink which a child takes when he is not ill contain the water and electrolytes which he needs (input). All drinks are mainly water and there is plenty of water in most food also. The main electrolytes (or salts) are sodium, potassium, chloride and bicarbonate. The body excretes water and electrolytes in the stools, in the urine and in the sweat (output). The kidney keeps the water and electrolytes in balance. If a lot of water is taken, a lot of water is passed in the urine. If there is an excess of any of the electrolytes in the body, the urine passes more of that electrolyte. In this way the amount of water and electrolytes in the blood and body fluids of a person keeps very much the same all the time, so long as the person is not ill.

Diarrhoea can upset this balance badly, especially in the child under 2 or 3 years of age. Not only is the child more likely to develop infection, because he has not met these infections before and so has not become immune, but simply because he is small, he has a small blood and body fluid volume, and cannot tolerate for long any serious disturbance in his fluid and electrolyte balance. In diarrhoea, the intestinal wall does not work normally; water and electrolytes pass from the bowel into the blood more slowly or not at all, and so they are passed in the stool. In some infections, water and electrolytes are positively excreted into the bowel instead of being absorbed. Thus the stool is loose and watery. This all results, if the diarrhoea is moderate or severe, in the output being greater than the input. This can be made worse by vomiting, and in fever there may be more liquid and salts lost in sweat also. The kidney tries to compensate by passing less urine (more concentrated because it still has to carry other waste products of the body), but its ability to do so is not enough and the child becomes dehydrated. Dehydration can occur gradually over several days, or if the diarrhoea is sudden and severe, it can happen quite quickly in a few hours.

In *moderate* dehydration the child will be passing only a small amount of urine; his eyes will appear sunken, as will the anterior fontanelle, if it is still open (infants); breathing and pulse will be faster than usual, mouth and tongue dry; but the most useful sign is that when the skin over the abdomen is pinched, the skinfold does not immediately go back to normal as it does in a normal child, but it takes several seconds to disappear. (This sign is not so reliable in children who are either obese or marasmic.)

In severe dehydration, all the above symptoms and signs are present, but to a greater degree. The child will not have passed urine at all for several hours. The eyes and fontanelle will be deeply sunken, breathing will be rapid and deep, the pulse rapid and very weak, perhaps even not able to be felt; the child will be very sleepy or unconscious, or having fits; and the skinfold when pinched up goes back very slowly. Unless rehydrated such a child is likely to die soon.

Even when the child with diarrhoea shows no sign of even moderate dehydration, it does not mean his state of hydration is normal. A child can lose fluids accounting for between 3 and 5 per cent of his usual body weight without showing any of the above signs at all. Moderate dehydration is accompanied by a deficit of fluids amounting to between 5 and 10 per cent of body weight; and the signs of severe dehydration as described above occur at a level of over 10 per cent. If reasonably accurate baby scales are available, weighing a child when he is brought for treatment of diarrhoea, although not essential, is a good idea. It is not done in order to have an idea of how much dehydration there is at that moment, because one rarely knows the previous day's weight. It is useful to have the weight then because, if the child is dehydrated, he should increase in weight when the dehydration is corrected. If the dehydration is getting worse, the weight will decrease.

Prevention and treatment of dehydration

The treatment of diarrhoeal disease has been greatly improved by the discovery that a solution of water and salts in certain proportions can be absorbed from the intestines into the bloodstream in diarrhoea (and the child can thus be *orally* rehydrated), even if there is vomiting, and even in spite of the active outpouring of fluid and electrolytes into the gut described above. However, for this to happen, the presence of glucose in the solution is essential, either as glucose or in the form of sucrose (common sugar), which is half glucose and half fructose. The most suitable solution is the one recommended by WHO and made from 1 litre of water plus a packet of ORS (Oral Rehydration Salts) containing 20 g of glucose, 3.5 g of sodium chloride, 2.5 g of sodium bicarbonate and 1.5 g of potassium chloride.* This should be given to every child under 3 with moderate or severe diarrhoea unless they need intravenous fluids (see below). Even if the child is not dehydrated, this solution, together with consumption of as much as possible of his normal fluid intake (especially breast milk), will prevent him from becoming so. If the child is mildly or moderately dehydrated,

*Some ORS packets are made with half of this amount, to be mixed with half the amount of water. The instructions on the packet must be read.

*Available from TALC, 30 Guildford Street, London WC1N 1EH, England.

this solution, plus as much of his usual intake as he will accept, will usually correct his dehydration. The child is to be given as much of the solution as he will take, but often, if he does not need it and has in fact no dehydration, he will not accept much. If the child is mildly or moderately dehydrated, he will be more thirsty and one should try to get him to take, in the first 4 or 5 hours, about 0.25 litre if he is under 6 months old, about 0.5 litre if 6–12 months, 0.5–0.75 litre if over 1 year and less than 3. For maintenance of hydration (in addition to as much of his usual fluids and diet as possible), about twice the above amounts is required during every 24 hours, according to age, until the diarrhoea is better. The child should preferably be fed the solution with a teaspoon, every few minutes.

The oral rehydration made with this solution is effective in 95 per cent of cases of acute diarrhoea, regardless of the causative micro-organism The mother is the one who should administer this solution, under supervision in the clinic for an hour or two, then at home. In spite of the fact that it has a sodium concentration of over 90 ml/litre, hypernatraemia need not be feared, although if the child's eyes become puffy (and this occasionally happens in infants under 6 months who have taken the solution well), plain water can be given for a few hours alternately with equal amounts of ORS solution.

Making a solution of salt and common sugar, with pinches of salt and a scoop of sugar (or better with a special measuring spoon*), is only partly effective, but it is much better than plain water when it is impossible to obtain ORS.

The child with any degree of dehydration less than severe can be rehydrated with ORS solution. If the child has severe dehydration and shock or is bordering on shock (pulse rapid and weak or unable to be felt, sleepy or unconscious, not passing urine for several hours) intravenous (i.v.) rehydration is needed. This means the child has to be sent to a hospital or a health centre specially equipped for i.v. rehydration. (Many children have died en route to hospitals which are far away.) There, Ringer's lactate solution is the most suitable commercially available solution (130 mmol sodium per litre,

4 mmol/l of potassium, 3 mmol/l of calcium, 109 mmol/l of chloride, 28 mmol/l of lactate) or a special 'Diarrhoea Treatment Solution' (117 mmol/l sodium, 13 mmol/l of potassium, 82 mmol/l of chloride, 48 mmol/l of lactate or acetate). Less suitable is half-strength Darrows (not enough sodium) and much less suitable are normal saline or half-normal saline in 5 per cent dextrose, or plain glucose or dextrose solutions. All these are for dire emergency use only, in the absence of either of the first two, and should be replaced by ORS solution as soon as the child is conscious.

Prevention of malnutrition following diarrhoeal disease

The second most important part of the treatment of diarrhoea is to prevent the worsening of the child's nutritional status. If the child is breast-fed, this should be continued during the diarrhoeal episode. Infants and children often have a poor appetite during an acute episode of diarrhoea, and what they do take of the usual fluid and semisolid diet may be less well absorbed than usual. It is most unhelpful to add to the problem by restricting the diet. Vomiting in diarrhoea is often the result of electrolyte imbalance, not of physical irritation by food or drink. There is no sound physiological reason to 'rest' the bowel. ORS solution is intended to be an *additional* input to make up for the additional output of diarrhoea or diarrhoea and vomiting: the fact that the child may vomit should not deter one from continuing to give the child ORS solution and to feed him his normal diet.

After the diarrhoea is over, the child should receive *extra* food to make up for the weight lost during the episode. The equivalent of one extra meal a day should be offered for about 2 weeks after the illness, but can be given better in the form of small frequent meals. Potassium-rich foods or drinks (fruit juice, bananas, coconut milk) may be particularly helpful. It is of interest that in all controlled trials the children treated with ORS gained weight much better for many months after the episode compared with children treated in what was then the usual way; but the reason for this quite definite favourable effect on nutrition remains unknown.

There is some place for antimicrobial drugs in treatment, but *not* routinely. The proper use of antimicrobials demands a precise diagnosis of the bacterial cause, and this is rarely practicable at primary health care level. For cholera, tetracycline is the most suitable, with furazolidine or erythromycin as alternatives. For shigella dysentery, ampicillin is the most useful, and for acute giardiasis, metronidazole. Neomycin should never be used in acute diarrhoea because it may damage the intestinal mucosa and contribute to malabsorption.

12
Parasites

Derrick B. Jelliffe and E.F. Patrice Jelliffe

Intestinal worms

The hookworm and the roundworm are the most important intestinal worms producing serious disease in tropical children, although in a few regions the tapeworm is common. The threadworm (pinworm), although frequently seen all over the world, is not considered here, as it is not a cause of important disease in children in the tropics.

Hookworm (*Ancylostoma duodenale, Necator americanus*)

These worms, which are about 2.5 cm long, live in the first part of the small intestine, especially the duodenum. Their heads are stuck into the wall of the intestine by means of hooks and they feed by sucking blood. Eggs are found in the stools and develop into active larvae, if faeces are passed on to warm, moist ground. The larvae can then rapidly penetrate any part of the human skin with which they come in contact. They then pass through the body and eventually reach the small intestine, where they grow into adult worms.

Disease picture

The main picture of hookworm disease is caused by prolonged loss of blood. The effect of hookworm infection depends on the number of worms present (and hence the amount of blood lost), and the nutrition of the child (especially as regards iron and protein).

A few hookworms in a fairly well-fed older child or adult produce no disease ('hookworm infection'), as the small blood loss can be replaced. However, in a young child, whose food lacks iron and protein, and who has high needs of these substances (as he is growing in size and also in the amount of blood his body contains), a large number of hookworms produce a slowly increasing anaemia ('hookworm disease'), mainly due to iron deficiency. If untreated, this eventually leads to death from heart failure.

The clinical picture is, then, of anaemia—weakness, pale conjunctiva, mucous membranes and palms, some swelling of the ankles, and ultimately heart failure.

Diagnosis

Three findings are needed to diagnose hookworm disease: (i) a definite anaemia, as shown by clinical examination (especially pale conjunctiva) and by a low haemoglobin, usually of below 40 per cent, (ii) many hookworm ova in the stools, and (iii) the presence of blood in the stools as shown by chemical test (positive occult blood test).

Treatment

1. *Anaemia.* If severe, a small intravenous blood transfusion, using sedimented red cells, may be given slowly, if the necessary skilled staff and apparatus are available (20 ml/kg or 10 ml/lb body wieght). If moderate, iron can be given by mouth (as ferrous sulphate mixture) or by intramuscular injection iron dextran (Imferon).

Deworm. Tetrachlorethylene (TCE) is cheap and effective (0.1 ml per kg body weight or 3/4 minim per lb body weight). It should be given in a liquid form on an empty stomach with no preliminary starvation or subsequent purgatives. It can be repeated daily for 3 days. If the haemoglobin is very low, it should preferably be raised to 40 per cent by transfusion or iron before deworming. If both roundworms and hookworms are present, the roundworms should be treated first, with piperazine (p.113), or drugs effective against both parasites should be given. These include bephenium, as a 1-day course of treatment for under 23 kg body weight 5g, and over 23 kg

10 g (divided into three doses), or mebendazole for 2–3 days (p.270). These have the disadvantage of being more expensive.

Prevention

Infection with the hookworm can be prevented: (i) by health education (p.190), so that mothers understand the way the disease is caught (and avoid allowing their children to walk on, and their babies to sit or lie on, contaminated soil); (ii) by the use of pit latrines; (iii) by the wearing of simple sandals (such as those made of old car tyres) or shoes by older children; and (iv) in some countries, by widespread 'deworming' campaigns.

Roundworm (*Ascaris lumbricoides*)

These large worms (20–25 cm long) live spread through the length of the intestine. Eggs are passed in the stools and may contaminate the ground or uncooked vegetables. If eggs are swallowed, adult worms develop in the small intestine, after various stages of development in the child.

Disease picture

A few roundworms in a well-fed child usually produce no ill effects, and are not noticed until a worm is either vomited by the child or passed in the stool, or a routine microscopic examination of the stool shows eggs to be present. Sometimes occasional mild abdominal pain, loose stools or vomiting may be produced.

Very occasionally, one or more roundworms may wander from the usual position in the small intestine. If it enters the bile ducts of the liver, jaundice or liver abscess will occur. If it reaches the stomach, it may be vomited. In the larynx, difficulty with breathing or even death from suffocation results; while, if roundworms enter the peritoneal cavity (by perforating the intestine), peritonitis occurs.

In heavy infections, obstruction can occur from a tangled ball of roundworms becoming stuck at the narrowest part of the intestine, that is where the small bowel enters the large intestine (i.e. ileocaecal junction). The child will be very ill, with signs of intestinal obstruction (i.e. vomiting, abdominal pain, intestinal distension, constipation). The round ball of worms sometimes may be felt through the abdominal wall.

In very heavy infections with up to hundreds of worms, these large parasites become dangerous nutritionally, especially in poorly fed, rapidly growing young children, as they use up a considerable portion of the food taken in by the child.

Treatment

Piperazine is used for the treatment of roundworm infections. It is given by mouth and paralyses the worms so that they are passed alive in the stools. No preparation or purgatives are needed. The dose is 2 g up to 2 years, 3 g for 2–5 years, 4 g over 5 years. As this drug has no side-effects in children and is cheap, it can be repeated on subsequent days, if required.

Tapeworms (*Taenia saginata* and *T. solium*)

Tapeworm infection occurs only from the eating of undercooked or raw beef or pork (in which animals, the 'intermediate stage' of the worm occurs). This worm is, therefore, only found commonly in a few groups of tropical children, such as the Masai of Kenya for whom underdone meat is a frequent food. In most communities, adult men get most of the meat, and most tropical children, in fact, have very little meat at all, and then usually well stewed.

Disease picture

Usually only one to three of these 50-cm long worms are present at a time and there are no complaints until the mother notices the flat, moving, white segments of worm, either in the stool or occasionally actually emerging from the child's anus.

Treatment

Mepacrine is often used, as it is safe and cheap. Eight tablets (1 tablet = 100 mg) are given for an older teenager, and four for a young child. One-quarter of the total number of tablets is given at 15-minute intervals. It has the disadvantage of sometimes producing vomiting. A saline purgative (such as magnesium sulphate) should be given 1 hour later.

Dichlorophen (Antiphen) is another drug used in the treatment of the tapeworm. The dose is 4–6 g given in a single dose by mouth on an empty stomach. No purgative is needed as dichlorophen has a laxative action. The drug digests the worm, so that parents should be told that the child will not pass identifiable segments.

Prevention

Tapeworm can be prevented easily if all beef and pork (including that of wild pig) is eaten only if fully cooked all through.

Filarial worms

Filarial worms are spread by the bites of various types of insects. There are three main types of filariasis affecting man.

1. *Flephantiasis.* This is due to blockage of lymph vessels (lymphatics) by filarial worms (*Wuchereria bancrofti*). The condition is uncommon in young children, but the huge swellings with thickened skin (elephantiasis) can be seen occasionally in school-age children. The leg or scrotum is most commonly affected. Surgical treatment may be required. Early infections may be treated with a course of Hetrazan (diethylcarbamazine).

2. *Onchocerciasis.* This infection is spread by the bite of a small black fly, sometimes called the buffalo gnat, which

breeds in fast-flowing streams. The infection is caused by the filarial worm *Onchocerca volvulus*, and occurs in some tropical areas of Africa and the Americas. The parasite lives in small round lumps (*Onchocerca* nodules) about 1–3 cm (½–1 inch) in size, lying beneath the skin. These are firm, painless, persistent and commonly found in the head, chest wall, knees or elbows.

The young forms (microfilariae) can enter the skin and produce a serious skin infection, which is persistent and very itchy. Affected skin is raised, thick, scaly and sometimes with patchy areas of lighter colour. This can be seen in older children.

The eyes may also be involved by microfilariae, even resulting in blindness. As this takes many years to develop, it usually only occurs in adults.

Diagnosis is confirmed by taking a small snip and examining it under the microscope for microfilariae.

Prevention may be attempted by spraying with DDT or, preferably, newer non-persistent insecticides (such as chlorphoxim), in the streams in populated areas where the flies breed. Treatment is by removing the nodules surgically, and by courses of diethylcarbamazine (Hetrazan) tablets.

3. *Loaiasis.* This filarial worm (*Loa loa*) only occurs commonly in parts of West Africa. It is spread by the bite of certain flies (*Chrysops*).

Symptoms are due to the adult worm wandering through the skin or over the eye. In the skin, painful, itchy, red swellings (known in West Africa as 'Calabar swellings') can occur. These may be several inches across, usually last for several days, and may be mistaken for osteomyelitis, especially if they occur in the region of a big joint.

In the eye, the worm is clearly visible as it passes across the front of the eye under the conjunctiva. There is a varying amount of pain and irritation.

Diagnosis is by the clinical picture (especially if the worm is visible in the eye) and by finding microfilariae in a blood flim.

Treatment is by removing adults if visible in front of the eye, and by courses of diethylcarbamazine (Hetrazan) tablets.

Schistosomiasis

There are three types of schistosomal worms, *Schistosoma mansoni*, *S. haematobium* and *S. japonicum*. With all of them, the disease is spread when urine or stools from an infected person is passed into water containing certain snails. The young parasites enter the snails and later are passed out into the water again. If they then come in contact with a person's skin, they are able to pass through it, enter the body and produce infection.

In all types of schistosomiasis, a rash, consisting of itchy red spots, can occur where the parasites enter the body, often in the feet or legs.

After some weeks or months, the main features of schistosomiasis occur, and these differ with the type according to the place where the parasite settles in the body. In *S. haematobium* infection, the worms live in the veins of the bladder so that haematuria (blood in the urine) is the first sign, often followed by increased frequency of passing urine accompanied by pain. In severe, prolonged infections, the bladder and ureters (leading from the bladder to the kidneys) may be permanently damaged or develop cancer.

In *S. mansoni* infections, the parasites are in the veins round the rectum (lower part of the large intestine). Blood and mucus appear in the stools and there may be diarrhoea. Again, if prolonged and severe, cancer can occur. In both of these types, the small constant loss of blood in either urine or stool can lead to anaemia; while cirrhosis of the liver (in which it becomes hard and shrunken) can occur.

S. japonicum is confined to parts of eastern Asia. It is the most severe type of infection. The worms live in the veins around the rectum, so that bloody diarrhoea occurs, but, in addition, eggs of the parasite are carried to the liver in large numbers and rapidly lead to cirrhosis, which is often fatal.

Diagnosis

The clinical picture is often suggestive, and can be confirmed by examining the stools or urine for eggs.

Prevention

Latrines should be available, to prevent infected persons from passing stools or urine into water. However, effective health education (p.190) to persuade people to use available latrines is very difficult. Snails (the necessary intermediate hosts for the parasites) may be attacked in various ways, as with special chemicals such as copper sulphate. People, especially schoolchildren, should be discouraged from bathing in possibly infected water, although this may be difficult if only a limited water supply is available locally. Early treatment is of value in decreasing the number of infected people in the area.

Treatment

The oldest treatment is with a course of injections of sodium antimony tartrate, intravenously, but this is not to be recommended. This is inexpensive, but toxic (poisonous) in some children. Instead, courses of intramuscular antimony compounds, such as lithium antimonylthiomalate (Anthiomaline), or various oral medicines, especially lucanthone (Miracil D) can be given.

Malaria

Malaria is common in many parts of the tropics. It is usually due to infection of the red blood cells with *Plasmodium falciparum* (MT malaria), and this is the main form of infection considered here. Malaria is spread from man to man by the bite of infected female anopheline mosquitoes. The parasites live in the red blood cells and destroy them, so that anaemia results.

Immunity

Immunity to infection with MT malaria varies under different circumstances.

Child Health in the Tropics

1. *Malaria continuous all year.* No infection occurs in young babies for 3–6 months or so, depending on the immunity they receive in the blood from their mothers while in the uterus. However, frequent, severe and sometimes fatal disease occurs in young children from 6 months to about 3 years of age, to be followed, if the child survives, by immunity in older children and adults, who may have a few malarial parasites in their blood but no actual disease, unless they are weakened by some other condition (i.e. such as some other illness, an operation or malnutrition).

2. *Malaria present only part of the year.* There will be less chance of repeated infections in childhood producing immunity, and so more severe effects of malaria may be expected in older children and adults.

3. *Malaria not usually present.* In mountainous regions, there may be no malaria as the anopheline mosquito may be unable to breed there. People from these parts, of all ages from early childhood to adult life, will have no immunity to malaria and may be expected to show severe disease, if they become infected (i.e. by moving into low-lying country where malaria does occur). The same occurs with expatriate (foreign) children and adults. It can also occur if malaria is reintroduced into an area from which the disease had previously been eradicated.

Disease picture

Severe malaria in the 6-month- to 3-year-old child in areas where malaria is present most of the year usually results in a weak, anaemic child, with a large spleen and liver, whose mother often reports frequent attacks of fever, bronchitis and loose stools. Cerebral malaria may develop, as a result of the blocking of the small blood vessels of the brain by red cells filled with malarial parasites, and is recognized by high fever, convulsions and unconsciousness. Even if treated early with chloroquine or quinine injections, cerebral malaria may still be followed by permanent brain damage, including mental deficiency and paralysis of a limb.

Older children with some immunity may have an occasional bout of fever, joint pains, headache etc., but, on the whole, show little sign of disease, except for an enlarged spleen.

Diagnosis

A positive blood slide for MT parasites and an enlarged spleen will be found, together, in severe cases, with some degree of anaemia. However, it may be difficult to tell the importance of the presence of a few parasites on the blood slide and the enlarged spleen as these may be present in very many children in heavily malarious areas. The complete picture of the particular child has to be taken into consideration. Blood slides that are very positive can usually be taken to indicate actual disease due to malaria.

Treatment

In areas where the malarial parasite is still sensitive, chloroquine, a 4–6 day course (1 tablet = 150 mg chloroquine), is usually recommended nowadays.

The treatment of malaria has become much more complicated in recent years, as parasites have developed which are less sensitive, or even resistant, to commonly used drugs, particularly to chloroquine. It is then important for the locally effective drug and its dosage to be known and used. If there is vomiting or the child appears very ill, the first dose may be given subcutaneously (5 mg/kg or 2.5 mg/lb body weight). The course by mouth is as follows:

up to 1 year	¼ tablet daily
1–5 years	½ tablet daily
5–10 years	1 tablet daily
10 years onwards	2 tablets daily

Suspected cases of cerebral malaria should be treated with an immediate chloroquine injection intramuscularly (or slowly and very dilute intravenously), 5 mg/kg or 2.5 mg/lb body weight, followed by a lumbar puncture (which will be clear in cerebral malaria, but will show cloudy fluid in meningitis), and by a thick-blood film (which will show a heavy infection with MT malaria parasites). The dosage of intramuscular chloroquine should be carefully calculated, and this route should only be used in cerebral malaria, or in other severe forms (e.g. rapidly developing anaemia).

Chloroquine should be given on the subsequent days by mouth, by gastric tube or by subcutaneous injection, according to the child's condition.

The dosage recommended may have to be varied in different parts of the world, as it seems likely that the malarial parasite varies in sensitivity to chloroquine. In some regions, more than the above dosage may be needed, while some treatment schedules use a 'loading dose' (e.g. double the regular dose) on the first day.

In countries where chloroquine resistance is usual (e.g. parts of South-east Asia), other drugs are necessary, such as quinine or one of the more recent drug combinations, such as Fansidar (pyrimethamine and sulphadoxine). Again, it must be stressed that *the best locally effective, least costly and simplest treatment needs to be known and used.*

If quinine is employed this can be cautiously given intravenously (10 mg/kg (5 mg/lb), very dilute or by drip) or intramuscularly (15 mg/kg; 7.5 mg/lb), as if for initial treatment in severe cases. For oral dosage, the following is suggested daily, divided into two or three doses, for at least 6 days:

up to 1 year	100–200 mg
1–3 years	200–300 mg
4–6 years	300–500 mg
7–11 years	500–1000 mg
12–15 years	1000–2000 mg

Prevention

Very large schemes of malaria prevention were carried out in the 1950s and later all over the world, usually by spraying the inside walls of houses with residual insecticides (such as DDT and others), so that anopheline mosquitoes were killed when they rest on them. Malaria was much reduced by this means in many countries, and apparently eliminated in some parts of the world, especially on islands. In large land areas, such as in Africa, problems of distance, roads, long, inaccessible frontiers and wars, have created great problems. Also in most regions of the world, malaria-carrying mosquitoes have become resistant to DDT and other commonly used insecticides. For this reason, together with the development of parasites which are resistant to chloroquine, rising costs and a lack of emphasis on what was mistakenly considered a solved problem, malaria is increasing in many areas and invading regions from which it had been eradicated. Recent preventive programmes have tried to combine the use of appropriate insecticides with older methods such as drainage, fish which eat mosquito larvae, etc.

Malaria can be prevented in non-immune children by the routine use of drugs to which the local form of the parasites is sensitive. This will usually be proguanil (Paludrine); ¼-1 tablet daily (1 tablet = 100 mg); or pyrimethamine (Daraprim) ¼-1 tablet weekly (1 tablet = 25 mg).

Whether to use drugs for all young children in areas where malaria is continuous is a difficult problem, as if this is done they may be prevented from developing immunity. Possibly this may be avoided by giving pyrimethamine or chloroquine fortnightly. Certainly, in children with repeated attacks of severe malaria, with malnutrition, or with some other illness, prompt treatment can be recommended, especially during the 'danger period' (p.65) between 6 months and 3 years, when malaria can add a serious additional burden to the child's nutrition.

In tropical regions where quartan malaria (due to *P. malariae*) or benign tertian malaria (due to *P. vivax*) occurs, special drugs, e.g. primaquine, may be needed, both in prevention and treatment, to destroy the persistent parasites which remain in the liver and produce relapses later.

Amoebiasis

Although human infection with *Entamoeba histolytica* occurs in most areas of the tropics, the frequency of human disease varies widely. In some parts of the tropics, clinical disease in children is a common and serious condition (e.g. South Africa, parts of India etc.).

Diarrhoea or dysentery

Commonly, *E. histolytica* infection occurs as diarrhoea with or without blood in the stools. There is no typical picture, and stool inspection may reveal a formed stool with just flecks of blood and mucus, or resembling redcurrent jelly. Amoebae can be seen by microscopic examination. In hospital circumstances, if the patient is co-operative, and if such stools are negative, gentle sigmoidoscopy with a child's sigmoidoscope may show ulceration of the large bowel, and in scrapings from such ulcers amoebae may be found. Varying degrees of fever, flatulence, large bowel colic, and pain in passing stools may occur.

Definite diagnosis mainly rests on finding the parasite. Repeated stool examinations may be necessary. Microscopic examination should always note the presence of red and white cells in fresh stool.

Patients with such symptoms must be treated. Flagyl (metronidazole) 24–40 mg in three divided doses daily for 5–7 days by mouth is the first line of treatment. However, amoebiasis varies considerably, and an alternative treatment needs to be considered, such as a 7-day course in tetracycline (p.274) or chloroquine (p.268).

Liver abscesses

This is usually uncommon and occurs when amoebae invade the liver. Children with liver abscess have fever and painful liver. If suspected, further hospital investigations are needed. Treatment is with metronidazole (p.271), and pus may have to be aspirated with a syringe.

Giardiasis

While not having the severe ill-effects of *E. histolytica*, infection with the microscopic parasite, *Giardia lamblia*, seems world wide, especially in less developed communities with poor hygiene. It is common in children and can be responsible for growth failure.

Infection is associated with decreased absorption of nutrients, passage of pale, frothy stools, and flatulence. Diagnosis is made by finding cysts in the stools. Sometimes, in cases of severe diarrhoea in small children, active moving forms can be seen in the stools.

As with *Entamoeba histolytica*, other symptoms are common, but this parasite should always be treated. Metronidazole is the drug of choice, in the same dosage as for amoebic diarrhoea. It has a cure rate of over 90 per cent. Only if this fails should mepracine, (quinacrine) be given in a dose of 5mg/kg daily in three divided doses for 10 days. This drug is not well tolerated by children because of its bitter taste.

13
Respiratory tract infections

Sa'ad Hijazi

For practical purposes, respiratory tract infections can be conveniently divided into three types, which may be called upper, middle and lower. It is necessary to do this because different methods of treatment are needed for each.

The function of the airway is primarily to transport gases to and from the air to the bloodstream. Oxygen must be taken in and carbon dioxide must be eliminated. Air breathed must be warmed and moistened, and harmful materials found in the air must be prevented from reaching the lungs. The upper part of the respiratory tract acts mainly as a filter, with active substances (lysozymes) in the nose helping to deal with harmful bacteria. The middle part of the respiratory tract makes up a combined air and food passage (pharynx). The surface of the respiratory tubes (bronchi) are covered with microscopic brush-like cilia, which remove inhaled particles.

The lower portion of the respiratory tract contains the alveoli (air sacs), surrounded by pulmonary blood vessels (capillaries), where gas exchange takes place.

A minimum number of 30 infections occur in the average individual from birth through adolescence, these occur mostly after the age of 3–6 months, when maternal antibodies decline in infants, as does the protective effect of breast-milk. This is also true in the first years of school, nursery school or day care centres.

Infants and children in tropical countries can demonstrate a pattern of clinical presentation which is somewhat different from what is reported in industrial countries, due to delay in reporting to the hospital and high frequency of associated malnutrition. All these result in a rather changed clinical picture which can affect the prognosis of the disease.

Hundreds of viruses have been demonstrated as causing respiratory tract infections. The most frequent bacteria are

124

the beta-haemolytic *Streptococcus, Heamophilus influenzae, Pneumococcus, Staphlyococcus* and *Meningococcus.*

Upper respiratory tract infections

The common cold

This is the most frequent paediatric illness in both tropical and temperate climates. A large number of viruses can be responsible. Some are unknown, some are known, such asrhinoviruses, adenoviruses etc. Its short incubation period extends from 12 to 72 hours; it is more common after the age of 6 months.

Symptoms are so familiar as not to need elaboration here. Coryza, sneezing, sore throat and tearing are the characteristics of simple common colds. Spread of infection to the paranasal sinuses can produce sinus headache, fever and purulent nasal discharge. Spread through the eustachian tubes (leading from the pharynx to the ears) can cause otitis media (infection of the middle ear). Spread down the respiratory tract may produce cough, hoarseness and respiratory stridor, and is termed laryngitis in older children and croup in younger ones. Further spread into the trachea and larger bronchi causes the persistent cough of tracheobronchitis.

Fever, if present, is seldom high in uncomplicated common colds. The mucous membranes of the nose and throat are infected. Otitis media and sinusitis are the most common complications of this condition, resulting from bacterial invasion.

If not complicated, the course of the illness is short, and complete recovery occurs after 3 to 7 days.

Treatment

No specific treatment is needed or available for the common cold, as it is a self-limiting disease. There is no justification for antibiotic treatment, as this does not prevent the common cold complications such as bronchitis, tracheitis or pneumonias. Aspirin or acetaminophen is helpful for fever.

In newborn and young infants, saline nose drops and suctioning with a bulb syringe will help if there is evidence of severe nasal congestion. Three drops are used in each nostril, with the patient lying flat on the back with the neck tilted backwards as far as is comfortably possible.

Recurrent rhinitis (chronic upper respiratory infection)

There are many children in the tropics who are not ill, but who have 'constant colds', with a watery discharge from the nose. They may sneeze frequently and cough at night-time, because of the discharge running back and irritating the throat.

The most common cause is repeated viral upper respiratory tract infection, although allergy may be responsible. The onset is usually after 6 months of age.

On examination, the lining of the nose is swollen and moist and the throat looks slightly red. Sometimes the tonsils are mildly inflamed and the neck glands are enlarged. The condition occurs more commonly during wet seasons.

Treatment

This mainly consists of reassurance. The parents can be told that their child's general health is good, as evidenced by adequate weight gain, and that the future outlook is good in that the number of 'colds' will decrease with time.

Acute pharyngitis and tonsillitis

Approximately 10 per cent of children with sore throat and fever have a streptococcal infection; 90 per cent have viral infections. Untreated streptococcal pharyngitis can result in acute rheumatic fever, glomerulonephritis, peritonsillar abscess (behind the tonsils), cervical adentitis (glands in the neck), otitis media and even septicaemia (spread of infection into the bloodstream). Vesicles (blisters) and ulcers are suggestive of viral infection; petechiae (small haemorrhagic spots) and a tonsillar exudate (whitish-yellow material on the tonsils) are suggestive of streptococcal infection. The only way to make a definitive diagnosis is by obtaining a throat culture, which is rarely possible.

Most children have a high temperature, feel generally unwell and have pain, especially on swallowing. On examination, there are enlarged, tender cervical lymph nodes, and red and inflamed tonsils.

Treatment

Virus infections will get better without antibiotics. The only treatment needed is rest, fluids by mouth and aspirin if fever is high (60–600 mg according to age). If the cause is due to group A beta-haemolytic *Streptococcus*, the drug of choice for the prevention of rheumatic fever — the most important complication of this infection — is either benzathine penicillin G given intramuscularly, or a 10-day course of oral penicillin. The intramuscular route ensures treatment for a sufficient length of time, while oral therapy is dependent upon the understanding and co-operation of the family and the patient.

Benzathine penicillin should be given as a single injection of 600 000–1 200 000 units, according to age. The dose for oral penicillin is 200 000–250 000 units three or four times a day for a full 10 days, even though temperature might return to normal.

For patients with histories of allergy to penicillin, oral erythromycin (30–50 mg/kg per day in three or four divided doses) or clindamycin (10–20 mg/kg per day in three or four divided doses) for 10 days is recommended. The sulphonamides, while effective in prophylaxis, are ineffective in the treatment of streptococcal infections.

Tonsils should not be removed for frequent tonsillitis, unless continuous preventive penicillin (200 000 units of penicillin G twice a day, or 250 mg phenoxymethylpenicillin twice a day, or benzathine penicillin 600 000 units every 2–3 weeks) for several months has failed to prevent frequent acute tonsillitis with fever; or because of persistent gross obstruction, recurrent peritonsillar abscess, recurrent pyogenic cervical adenitis, and some cases of recurrent otitis media.

Otitis media

Infection of the middle ear is a common complication of upper respiratory diseases and allergic rhinitis in infants and young children. Short episodes of eustachian tube obstruction (the tube connecting the middle ear with the back of the throat), can occur in the absence of middle ear infection. If the blockage is not relieved, pus may be formed which may burst through the ear drum, leaving a hole (perforation), or even lead to severe infection of the mastoid bone (behind the ear), causing mastoiditis.

Disease picture

Otitis media is common in the tropics but is not often recognized until the child's mother notices pus discharging from the ear. For the child too young to talk, the only clue will be behaviour. The infant may just be very fussy, or cry when swallowing. There may be pulling or rubbing of the affected ear. Examination with an auroscope shows a general redness of the ear drum, with some bulging or fullness. If proper treatment is started, the otitis will not progress beyond this stage, but will subside, leaving a normal ear drum.

Treatment

The use of 0.5 per cent ephedrine nose drops with the head tilted backwards will help to maintain an adequate airway, and to shrink the tissues at the opening of the eustachian tube. Aspirin should be given to reduce the discomfort and fever. A combination of ephedrine or pseudo-ephedrine, elixir of phenylephrine (Neosynephrine), or syrup of phenylpropanolamine hydrochloride (Propadrine) and syrup of an anti-histaminic, may be of value. For most children, procaine penicillin, 400 000 units given daily by intrasmuscular injection for 5–10 days, is sufficient. Long-acting benzathine penicillin is also effective. Penicillin with triple sulphonamide or ampicillin alone is preferred in children less than 4 years of age, or for those proved by bacterial culture to be infected with *H. influenzae.* Very occasionally, the ear drum must be incised (myringotomy) to release pus.

Children who have repeated attacks of otitis media or chronic ear infection should be advised to keep water out of the ears by plugging them with cotton soaked in mineral oil when washing or bathing. Swimming should be forbidden. Repair of the ear drum may need to be done at about age 10 or older, if rupture of the drum has occurred earlier. If no proper treatment is given, hearing loss, or even brain abscess, meningitis or mastoiditis may occur.

Mid-respiratory tract infection

Laryngotracheobronchitis (croup)

Two common forms of croup exist: an acute laryngotracheobronchitis causing progressive hoarseness, cough and inspiratory stridor (noisy breathing), and a spasmodic variety occurring together with upper respiratory infection or allergy. In spasmodic croup, the hoarseness and stridor are abrupt in onset and tend to disappear rapidly.

The typical picture of croup is familiar to all responsible for the health care of children. A brassy cough, hoarseness, inspiratory stridor, and flaring of the nostrils are characteristic, and occur most severely at night.

The more severely ill child may be cyanotic, restless and have a rapid pulse. After a prolonged bout of croup, the patient may become exhausted. In this case, tracheostomy (opening the trachea) must be seriously considered.

Most patients who have no inspiratory stridor at rest may be treated at home. The parents should be instructed about the signs and symptoms of increased airway obstruction. If feasible, cool mist can be helpful in the home treatment for mild croup. Fluid replacement and maintenance must be provided, preferably by mouth (p.106). In the case of a severely ill child, this may have to be done by the intravenous route. If available, 25–30 per cent oxygen is often administered. A brief course of 0.5 mg/kg per day of dexamethasone or a comparable agent in four divided doses for 1–3 days may be beneficial in cases of severe croup. Antibiotics are useful when a bacterial organism, such as *H. influenzae*, is responsible.

Particularly severe is the croup caused by *H. influenzae* type B, causing epiglottitis, which is a severe, life-threatening inflammation of the epiglottis (thin end of the soft palate). Symptoms are abrupt in onset and include inspiratory stridor, difficulty or inability to speak, fever and a very sick appearance. A bright cherry-red epiglottis confirms the diagnosis. With epiglottitis, there is a great danger of complete laryngeal obstruction, occurring abruptly. Immediate hospitalization and the availability of a physician to perform tracheostomy are indicated, wherever possible, as at least 50 per cent of children with epiglottitis will require tracheostomy. Ampicillin (intramuscularly or intravenously) and cold steam vaporization should be initiated, when feasible.

Lower respiratory tract infection

Bronchitis

This is usually an extension of a cold or of an upper respiratory infection and has many of the same symptoms as pneumonia: cough, fever and labored breathing. Asthmatic bronchitis is a somewhat imprecise term for the wheezing and cough which occur in allergic children who have similar symptoms.

Bronchitis may be acute or chronic, infectious (viral, bacterial, etc.), or due to chemical or mechanical irritation of the bronchial epithelium.

Clinical picture

Bronchitis nearly always follows a cold. There is a dry non-productive cough for the first 4–6 days, after which the cough is likely to become productive with yellow sputum (although this may be swallowed in younger children). Low-grade fever may be present. Chest pain aggravated by cough may develop. After 10 days, mucus production decreases and the cough gradually disappears.

Treatment

The ideal treatment for all types of bronchitis includes postural drainage and chest percussion preceded by bronchodilator inhalation, if these are available (which will not usually be the case in developing countries). Expectorants have no proved benefit. Cough suppressants are not indicated since coughing is necessary to clear secretions. Mist or high humidity often reduce the symptoms. Broad-spectrum antibiotics should be used in bronchitis due to bacterial infection.

Acute bronchiolitis

This is an acute and potentially serious disease which occurs during colder weather in children below the age of 2 years. Respiratory syncytial virus (RSV) is the most frequent causative organism, but other viruses can give the same picture.

Disease picture

All patients with bronchiolitis have some degree of oxygen lack and cyanosis (blueness), which may become severe.

Rhinitis (infected nose), cough, expiratory wheezes and a rapid pulse are the main characteristics of the condition.

Treatment

Admission to hospital is recommended for infants with bronchiolitis who are less than 2 months of age or for those who have cyanosis and wheezing. The inspired gas should be moistened (humidified) and enriched with oxygen, when appropriate apparatus is available. Achieving and maintaining a state of normal hydration are essential, and oral rehydration fluids can be used (p.106). A trial treatment with epinephrine 1 : 1000 solution, 0.01 ml/kg subcutaneously, with or without theophylline, 2–4 mg/kg orally every 6 hours, can be undertaken.

In more severe cases, broad-spectrum antibiotic therapy is indicated, especially if a secondary bacterial infection is suspected. There is no evidence that corticosteroids influence the course of the disease. Sedation should not be used unless the patient is intubated (with a tube through the larynx to the lungs) and receiving assisted ventilation, which will only be possible in some large hospitals.

Pneumonia

Pneumonia usually results from a spread of infection downward from the nose and throat. The majority of acute pneumonias are viral in origin, and frequently remain undiagnosed as the disease is often subclinical or mild. The incidence of bacterial pneumonias is about one-third of all acute infections of the lower respiratory tract. These are more serious in nature and are seen most frequently in hospitals.

Pneumonias are either bacterial or non-bacterial. Bacterial pneumonias are best classified by the organism responsible rather than by anatomical distribution (eg. lobar or bronchopneumonia), since the antibiotic therapy to be used depends on an exact (or probable) knowledge of the particular organism responsible.

Bacterial pneumonia

Disease picture   The onset is usually rapid and often follows an upper respiratory infection. Fever and a rapid heart rate are the most important findings. Cough in infants below the age of 6 weeks of age can be very suggestive of pneumonia. Older children may complain of chest or abdominal pain. Abnormal physical findings in the chest may precede x-ray abnormalities.

Pneumococci are the most common cause of bacterial pneumonia. *Haemophilus influenzae* can cause a similar clinical picture, but may not respond to penicillin alone. Pneumonia caused by group A beta-haemolytic streptococci is uncommon, but can be severe. Staphylococcal infection has a special tendency to produce small lung abscesses. Tuberculosis should be considered if pneumonia does not respond to usual antibiotic treatment.

Treatment   The need for admission to hospital depends on the severity and age of the case, and on space in the wards, distance etc. Antibiotics should be selected on the basis of the clinical presentation and probable organism responsible. Penicillin is the drug of choice for pneumonia due to *Streptococcus pneumoniae*, group A streptococci, and penicillin-sensitive staphylococci. Ampicillin should be used in *H. influenzae* pneumonia. In resistant staphylococcal infections, intravenous sodium methicillin or nafcillin should be used. In most circumstances, bacterial culture will not be available. In this case, treatment will probably be started with penicillin, and moved to other antibiotics if a rapid response does not occur.

Supportive measures such as humidified oxygen, pulmonary physiotherapy and intravenous fluids are indicated in some severe cases, if these are available.

Viral pneumonia

This is a relatively common and potentially serious disease, particularly in infants, as it involves both the conducting airways (bronchi) and the alveoli. The onset is preceded by an upper respiratory infection with slower progression than with pneumonia due to bacteria.

Treatment consists of humidifed oxygen and pulmonary physiotherapy, if available. Antibiotics are indicated if a secondary bacterial infection is suspected, and will often be needed as, in most developing countries, histories may be uncertain and bacterial investigation unavailable.

14
Tuberculosis

Nimrod Bwibo

Tuberculosis is a common infectious disease in the tropics. This is largely due to overcrowding, poverty, malnutrition and a high prevalence of other infectious diseases.

Tuberculosis of the lung (pulmonary tuberculosis) is the commonest form of this disease. Infections outside the lung (non-pulmonary infections) also occur frequently.

Tuberculosis is caused by bacteria called *Mycobacterium tuberculosis*, of which there are many types. The commonest type causing disease in man is the human variety, followed by the bovine type. This bacteria is usually spread from person to person through inhalation of airborne bacilli in droplet form. The source of infection is usually an adult with 'open' pulmonary tuberculosis with cavities in the lungs. Such a patient coughs out tuberculosis bacilli into the air. Children do not normally have 'open' pulmonary tuberculosis, and thus do not cough out these bacteria. Children are, therefore, infected by adults and not by other children. Children can also be infected by the bovine type of the bacteria, when they drink infected milk from cows with tuberculosis.

Pulmonary tuberculosis

Following an infection with tubercule bacilli, children develop 'primary tuberculosis', usually in the lungs. The main feature of primary pulmonary tuberculosis is an enlargement of lymph glands at the root of the lung (hilar lymph glands). These glands are found where the trachea divides to form the two bronchi. Lymph glands along the trachea (paratracheal glands) may also enlarge. The enlarged glands may press on the trachea and/or bronchi, causing a partial block, thus interfering with air entering and leaving the lungs.

In most cases these glands heal, leaving the child with some

135

immunity to the disease. Such a child shows a positive tuberculin test. Healed glands may lay down calcium (calcify) after many months or several years. These can usually be seen in x-rays of the chest. However, calcification does not imply complete healing as the disease may become active again under certain conditions.

Another feature of primary pulmonary tuberculosis is the 'primary focus' (original site of infection). This is usually at the edge of the lung and may also heal with calcification.

Sometimes the gland (and, rarely, the primary focus) progresses to form tuberculous pus (caseation) within its centre. The disease then spreads, particularly in very young children, in the poorly nourished and the debilitated. The caseous material (tuberculosis 'pus') may burst into a bronchus, scattering infection into other parts of the lung. Alternatively, a gland leaks its contents into a blood vessel, spreading the disease: (i) throughout the lung as miliary tuberculosis (so called because small areas of infection about the size of millet seeds are scattered in the lungs); or (ii) to such distant parts as the meninges, bone, kidneys, spleen and liver.

Rapid progression of the disease may follow measles or whooping cough. A child who fails to improve after an attack of these infections should be suspected of having pulmonary tuberculosis.

Disease picture

There is nothing absolutely diagnostic about the clinical picture of childhood tuberculosis. Rather, some points in the history and physical examination arouse suspicion. These, in combination with results of special investigations, help one to arrive at a diagnosis.

History of contact

There may be a history of contact with an adult with chronic cough, coughing up blood (haemoptysis) or with proven tuberculosis. A history of contact with one who died with the above features should also be very important. A negative history may be given, even though there is actually a relative with these symptoms. A repeat history, taken when the parents are used to the health worker, may give additional information. It is also important to ask for a history of chronic cough in the *ayahs* (nannies) or other servants.

Symptoms

There may be no symptoms in infected children. As said before, these children may have a positive tuberculin test as the only indication that they have been infected.

Tuberculosis is a chronic disease. A child with the disease who has symptoms has usually been suffering for more than a few weeks with any of the following symptoms.

Cough

This is a common symptom and may be of any sort (e.g. productive and loose, or dry and barking). The cough is very persistent and may be similar to whooping cough. There may be wheezing like asthma. Other causes of chronic cough, such as asthma or inhaled foreign body, should be kept in mind. Normally, the child swallows the sputum and does not cough it out.

Shortness of breath (dyspnoea)

This is more usually caused if infection involves a considerable part of the lung, or if a pleural effusion (fluid in the pleural cavity) occurs.

Fever

There is usually a low-grade fever, which may be intermittent, being present any time of the day, but more commonly occurring in the evening and night. A high fever persisting for a long time with no obvious cause, such as malaria or typhoid, should lead one to suspect tuberculosis.

Poor appetite

These children have poor appetite, and, as their food intake is low and their infection increases their needs, they fail to thrive and lose weight.

Fatigue

These children are less energetic and less playful. The combination of these symptoms—fever, cough, loss of weight and poor appetite—should arouse suspicion of tuberculosis in any child in the tropical countries. Another area of suspicion is a child with pneumonia which fails to improve on effective antibiotics; and a child who fails to improve after measles or whooping cough and continues to have the above symptoms.

Signs

Fever

A temperature chart shows continuous low-grade fever or intermittent fever. There may be persistent high fever.

Marasmus or severe wasting

Children may seek treatment when the disease is advanced. Such children may present with features of malnutrition, such as marasmus or even kwashiorkor (p.66).

Pulmonary signs

There may be no pulmonary signs. Positive signs are crepitation (cracking sounds heard through the stethoscope), either only in the diseased area or scattered in the case of widespread pulmonary disease. Rhonchi (wheezing sounds heard through the stethoscope) may be present when a gland is pressing a bronchus. A dull percussion note is found when there is pleural effusion or consolidation.

Non-pulmonary tuberculosis (tuberculous adenitis)

Tuberculosis is the commonest cause of enlargement of the neck gland in children in tropical countries. Initially, the glands are painless and separately enlarged. As they enlarge further, they become soft and stick together. They may develop sinuses,which discharge onto the skin. This infection is almost always due to the human type of tubercle bacilli, but can, rarely, be due to bovine bacilli acquired from milk.

Other lymph glands may also be affected, for example those in the axilla (underarm) and groin. Causes of lymph node enlargement like pyogenic adenitis (due to bacterial infection), leukaemia, lymphoma and Hodgkins disease are important differential diagnoses.

Tuberculous meningitis

This is infection of membranes covering the brain (meninges) and is usually a complication of primary tuberculosis. It occurs more frequently in infants and in early childhood, 3 to 6 months after a primary infection. It may occur after measles.

Tuberculous meningitis is usually of slow onset, presenting for many weeks with general non-specific symptoms of ill-health. These symptoms progress to features of meningeal irritation, characterized by headache and pain at the back of the neck, and to severe symptoms of vomiting, convulsions, drowsiness, and coma.

Diagnosis in the early stage is difficult. In advanced disease, the patient has stiffness of the neck and arching of the back. Confirmation of the diagnosis is based on examination of cerebrospinal fluid obtained by lumbar puncture. This has characteristic changes in cells, sugar and elevated protein. Rarely does one demonstrate tubercle bacilli or grow them on culture.

Tuberculous meningitis carries a poor prognosis (outlook).

Mortality is high and the survivors have severe neurological complications. Early diagnosis and early starting of drug therapy are helpful.

Bone and joint tuberculosis

Tuberculosis of the bone and joints results from bloodstream spread of tubercle bacilli from a lung lesion. Only rarely does it result from drinking unboiled milk containing tubercle bacilli from infected cows. The disease comes on many years after the pulmonary infection.

The spine is the commonest bone to be involved. Here, the disease destroys one or more vertebrae, usually in the thoracic region, leading to angulation deformity of the vertebral column (Pott's disease). Caseous material (thick tuberculous pus) from the destroyed vertebrae forms an abscess (paravertebral abscess) which may press on the spinal cord causing neurological symptoms: weakness in the lower limbs and eventually paralysis (paraplegia). This is usually associated with bladder dysfunction (such as inability to control micturition). X-ray of the affected area of the spine shows collapsed vertebrae with a paravertebral abscess.

Joint tuberculosis affects the large joints and rarely the smaller ones. The hip and knee are commonly affected. There is a slow onset of swelling, slight warmth and slight pain, with increasing deformity at the affected joint. These features are unlike those of pyogenic arthritis (infection with other bacteria), which are accompanied by rapid swelling with much pain and high fever.

X-ray of the involved joint shows narrowing of the joint space, and osteoporosis (loss of calcium) of the adjacent bone. There may be obvious destruction of the ends of the bone with fusion of the joint.

Other forms of extra-pulmonary tuberculosis occur, for example: abdominal tuberculosis, tuberculosis of the kidneys, tuberculosis of the eye and skin, but space does not allow their description.

Investigations

The following investigations are used for the diagonsis of tuberculosis.

Tuberculin skin tests

In these tests, a small amount of specially prepared solution (tuberculin) from tubercle bacilli is used. There are two forms of tuberculin—Old Tuberculin (OT) and Purified Protein Derivative (PPD)—which are injected into the skin in the Mantoux test or Heaf test.

In a Mantoux test, 0.1 ml of the tuberculin is injected into the skin (intradermally) using a Mantoux syringe—0.1 ml contains one tuberculin unit (1 TU). Stronger solutions of 5 TU may be used. In the case of the Heaf test, tuberculin is applied on the skin and injected into the skin by a special puncture apparatus (Heaf gun).

The results of tests are read after 72 hours. In the case of the Mantoux test, an induration of the skin at the site of injection is read by measuring the diameter of the induration, and the results are scored as follows.

No induration or induration less than 5 mm	Negative
Induration 5–9 mm	Doubtful
Induration 10–14 mm	1 (+)
Induration 15–20 mm	2 (+ +)
Induration 20–30 mm	3 (+ + +)
Induration above 30 mm or ulceration	4 (+ + + +)

In the case of the Heaf test, the results are scored as follows.

No marks	Negative
Four or more prongs	1 (+)
Ringed prongs, normal centre	2 (+ +)
Ringed prongs and raised centre	3 (+ + +)
Ulcerated lesion	4 (+ + + +)

Tuberculin tests may be negative because of a poor technique or use of out-of-date tuberculin. Tuberculin deteriorates quickly in warm climates, hence it should be prepared fresh. Where the technique and tuberculin material are satisfactory, the test may be negative in the presence of an active disease when there is malnutrition, or with an overwhelming disease like tuberculous meningitis or miliary tuberculosis, or when there has been a recent infectious disease, such as measles or whooping cough.

A strongly positive tuberculin test under 2 years of age should be regarded by itself as proof that there is an active disease, and the child should be treated.

X-ray of chest

Where it is possible to carry out a chest x-ray, useful information can be obtained concerning pulmonary tuberculosis. Chest x-rays may show nothing, especially in the early stages of the disease. Otherwise, the x-ray shows enlarged hilar glands, or areas of lung consolidation, or miliary mottling, or pleural effusion, depending on the spread in the lungs. There may be a combination of these features. It is difficult to distinguish consolidation due to tuberculosis from that to ordinary pneumonia. X-ray findings in bone and joint tuberculosis have been explained above.

Sputum examination

In infants and young children, sputum is not available as these children cough and swallow it. It is necessary to do gastric washouts in the morning to obtain this swallowed sputum for examination. This requires admission to hospital and a laboratory capable of carrying out this test. A deep laryngeal swab may obtain coughed up sputum from the larynx for examination. Older children may readily produce sputum. From any of these sources, the sputum is examined by staining for tubercle bacilli, and what are seen are called acid-fast bacilli for culture, the sputum is cultured for

Mycobacterium tuberculosis. The results take a long time and the positive cultures are few and with few bacteria grown.

Investigation of family

Inquiry should be made of contact with an adult with tuberculosis or with symptoms suggesting tuberculosis. X-ray of such an adult can be very useful in revealing pulmonary tuberculosis with cavities. Other children who are similarly exposed to the same adult should be investigated for tuberculosis. In practice, it is better to examine all children in the household.

Treatment of tuberculosis

It is better to diagnose tuberculosis early and start effective drug therapy as soon as possible. This ensures a high cure rate and lessens the chance of the disease spreading in the body.

General management

The child should receive a generous nutritious diet containing all nutrients, including calories, protein, vitamins and minerals. The child should have adequate rest and sleep. Other medical problems are looked for and treated, including anaemia (p.83), malnutrition (p.65), and parasitic infestations (p.110).

Drug therapy

Three drugs are commonly used in the management of tuberculosis in childhood: Streptomycin, isonicotinic acid hydrazide (INH) and thiacetazone (or para-aminosalicylic acid—PAS). Newer drugs may be used where there is resistance to these primary drugs.

Streptomycin

This is given as a single daily intramuscular injection of 20–40 mg/kg (10-20 mg/lb) body weight for 1 month. This usually requires hospital admission for injections.

INH or INAH (isonicotinic acid hydrazide)

This is given as a single daily dose of 10–20 mg/kg (5–10 mg/lb) body weight. Children normally tolerate it well. It is the most effective drug against tuberculosis. Higher doses are given for miliary spread, tuberculous meningitis and bone disease. For tuberculous meningitis, one can start with even higher doses of 30 mg/kg for the first few weeks. This drug is continued for 12–18 months, depending upon the severity of the disease. Treatment may be extended to 24 months in tuberculous meningitis.

Thiacetazone (TbI)

This is administered in a dose of 3–5 mg/kg (1.5–2.5 mg/lb) body weight, with a maximum of 200 mg per day.

INH and thiacetazone are sometimes given in a combined tablet (Thiazina). The proportion of INH and thiacetazone in Thiazina should be checked in each area where it is used. In East Africa, each tablet contains 100 mg INH and 50 mg thiacetazone. This satisfies the total amount of thiacetazone the child requires, but INH is normally supplemented to reach the dosages mentioned above. One tablet of INH contains 50 mg. The dosage schedule for Thiazina is shown in Table 14.1.

Table 14.1 Dosage schedule for Thiazina

Body Weight (kg)	Thiazina tablets
0–1	½
11–20	1
21–30	2
Above 30	3

PAS (para-aminosalicylic acid)

This is administered as 200 mg/kg (100 mg/lb) body weight daily in the form of a solution or powder. The drug is divided into three doses a day, and is given orally. It is an unpleasant drug and children refuse to take it; it causes vomiting. It has been replaced by thiacetazone in most centres.

Corticosteroids

In some centres, corticosteroids are given in selected cases with much benefit. They are given as prednisolone 0.5 mg/kg (0.25 mg/lb) body weight orally. Their value in tuberculous meningitis is to improve appetite and to reduce adhesions, thus enabling other drugs to reach the infected areas.

It is important to stress to the parents that tubercle bacilli take a long time to be eliminated by the drugs, so that treatment has to be continued regularly for a long time. The default rate is high and parents may stop giving medicine and bringing the child for follow-up, thinking the child is cured when symptoms like cough and fever cease.

For bone and joint disease, besides drug therapy, orthopaedic management is required. A plaster jacket is required for resting the spine, and a paravertebral abscess may need draining. In the case of knee or hip infection, bedrest is given, and traction is applied on the affected joint. A special plaster can also be used and the patient treated at home. An operation to fuse the joint is done when the joint is grossly destroyed in older children.

Response to treatment

This is usually slow. Improvement in appetite, fall in temperature, and weight gain are the features of healing disease. X-ray changes take a long time to improve. Neck glands decrease in size during therapy, but have been known to enlarge during early therapy.

Prevention of tuberculosis

As with any other disease, prevention is better than cure. This is more so with tuberculosis, a disease that takes many months to treat. In considering prevention, one should remember that the child gets tuberculosis from an adult with open lung disease, and rarely from cow's milk. The various methods of prevention fall into two categories.

Decreasing the chance of infection

This requires improvement in the standard of living, including provision of a well ventilated house with reduced chances of overcrowding. Adults with open tuberculosis should be isolated while undergoing treatment, and should use sputum containers for spitting—however simple these may be. These can be burnt or buried at the end of each day. Careless spitting should be discouraged. The mouth should be covered as the patient coughs. Surveys should be conducted in the community for case-finding.

The newborn babies of mothers with tuberculosis are at great risk of contracting the disease from their mothers. However, the baby should not be separated from the mother as the danger of suffering from malnutrition when there is no breast-feeding is a serious risk. In such a situation, the baby is given prophylactic INH, 20 mg/kg (10 mg/lb) body weight daily for 6 months, and, at the same time, the mother must continue her treatment. At the end of the period, the drug is stopped and the baby is given BCG vaccination. The mother should no longer have bacilli in her sputum by this time. If the baby is infected then full therapy is instituted. Pasteurization of milk or boiling milk kills any *Mycobacterium tuberculosis* and is an effective way of reducing the chance of infection from milk of infected cows.

Increasing resistance

General resistance to tuberculosis is increased by good nutrition—emphasizing the need for sound young-child feeding (p.52). Weakening diseases like anaemia (p.83), malaria (p.117), and other parasitic diseases (p.110) should be treated. Prevention of measles and whooping cough by effective immunization (p.201) is also very important.

Immunization against tuberculosis with BCG should be done at birth and repeated at the age of 12–14 years. BCG vaccination is a safe method. It contains a suspension of tubercle bacilli which have been specially treated so that they no longer cause disease. Immunity acquired from BCG is limited and does not stop an infant from getting tuberculosis. Hence, this precaution should be taken together with the others.

Vaccination with BCG is normally given to Mantoux-negative individuals, a requirement which is not looked for in the newborn. Children with positive Mantoux may have been exposed to tuberculosis and should be investigated.

In some countries, particularly India, the Mantoux test has not been required before BCG vaccination. Direct BCG is given, and those children with accelerated BCG reactions are presumed to have tuberculosis and are investigated for it.

15

Infections of the nervous system

John Vince and John Biddulph

Meningitis

Meningitis is inflammation of the meninges, the membranes that cover the brain and spinal cord.

Acute bacterial meningitis

This is the most common type of meningitis and occurs throughout the world, with a high incidence in many tropical countries. It can occur in any age group, but most commonly in the first few years of life. The organisms usually involved in children are *Haemophilus influenzae*, *Streptococcus pneumoniae*, (pneumococcus) or *Neisseria meningitidis* (meningococcus). Meningococcal meningitis may occur in epidemics.

Intestinal (Gram-negative) bacteria are often responsible for meningitis in newborn babies, who are also sometimes infected by organisms which are harmless in older children. In children with sickle-cell disease and those whose body defences against infection are lowered, meningitis may be caused by a wide variety of bacteria.

Infection usually enters the body through the respiratory tract and reaches the brain through the bloodstream. There may be signs of infection in the respiratory tract (pneumonia or sore throat), but more often there are not. Sometimes, however, the infection may spread into the meninges from a nearby infected area, such as otitis media (p.128) and mastoiditis (p.128), or through a skull fracture. Occasionally, infection may be introduced by an unsterile lumbar puncture, or may enter through a congenital defect such as spina bifida.

Disease picture

This depends on the patient's age. It is important to:

1. remember that symptoms of meningitis in babies and young children are non-specific, and there are often no definite signs; and therefore

2. think of meningitis with every sick baby and child.

In this way, meningitis will be diagnosed and treated early.

In neonates (babies up to 28 days old). The most important symptom is failure to suck. Other symptoms which may be present are a high-pitched cry, being either very irritable or very quiet, and vomiting. Fits and cyanotic attacks should always suggest the possibility of meningitis. Signs may be completely absent. There may be fever but, quite often, particularly in small babies, the temperature may be normal or low.

If present, a bulging fontanelle is a helpful sign, but often the fontanelle is normal. Jaundice may be present. Sometimes the only sign may be that the baby 'doesn't look well'.

In children up to 2 years old. Symptoms and signs are again non-specific. There is usually a history of fever and irritability, poor feeding, and sometimes vomiting. A high-pitched irritable cry may be present. Parents may say that the child has been staring. The child may turn his head away from the light (photophobia). Fits always suggest the possibility of meningitis. On examination, affected children usually have a fever. They may be either irritable or quiet. A worried or staring expression is often present. The child *may* have a stiff neck and *may* have pain when the hip is flexed and the knee straightened (a positive Kernig's sign). Bulging of the fontanelle (if still open) *may* be present. These three signs—neck stiffness, Kernig's sign and a bulging fontanelle—are helpful *if* they are present. They are, however, often absent.

In children over 2 years old. The non-specific symptoms found in younger children are usually present, and the child often complains of severe headache. In severe cases the child may be confused or unconscious. Neck stiffness and a positive Kernig's sign are found more frequently than in younger children, but are not always present. In advanced meningitis at any age, neurological abnormalities such as paralysis of limbs, eyes or face may be found.

Signs in other parts of the body. It should be remembered that, although meningitis most often occurs by itself, it sometimes occurs with pneumonia, when the child will have signs of this illness. Children with meningitis caused by meningococcus may have pain and swelling in the joints (arthritis). Bleeding spots in the skin (purpura) may occur in severe meningitis.

Meningism is the term given to pain and neck stiffness on bending the neck forwards. It is often present in older children with meningitis, but it is also sometimes found in children with other febrile illnesses such as pneumonia, otitis media and malaria. The presence of meningism is almost always an indication to do a lumbar puncture for cerebrospinal fluid examination so that meningitis, if present, can be diagnosed.

Diagnosis

Delayed diagnosis and inadequate treatment may have severe consequences. Since meningitis can only be diagnosed with certainty by an examination of the cerebrospinal fluid, (CSF), *lumbar puncture (LP) should be performed in all children suspected of having meningitis.*

All cerebrospinal fluid specimens should be examined under the microscope, because fluid which looks clear to the eye may contain a significant number of cells. In bacterial meningitis, many pus cells are present. Gram-staining may reveal bacteria, and bacteria may grow on culture. The protein level is usually raised and the sugar level is usually low. In early bacterial meningitis, or when the child has already received antibiotics, the cell count may be low and the bacteria may neither be seen nor cultured.

In cases where lumbar puncture is unsuccessful *or* where interpretation of cerebrospinal fluid findings is difficult, a diagnosis of bacterial meningitis should be assumed and full treatment given.

Treatment

Treatment should be started as soon as possible. If it is not possible to do an LP, and there is likely to be a delay between the time the child is suspected of having meningitis and the time he can be admitted to health centre or hospital, treatment should be started immediately.

The child should always be weighed to allow calculation of correct drug dose.

Antibiotics. The choice of antibiotic depends on the sensitivity of the usual organisms and the availability of suitable drugs.

Chloramphenicol is the best single antibiotic agent, since it is usually effective against the common causative organisms.

In children older than 1 month, chloramphenicol should be given in a dose of 25 mg/kg intramuscularly, 6-hourly. Intravenous administration is not necessary and should only be given if the child is receiving intravenous fluids for correction of dehydration. When the child has improved, as shown by a normal temperature and a return to eating and drinking, chloramphenicol may be given orally, except in young infants in whom continued intramuscular administration is more reliable.

Penicillin G is also widely used, usually together with chloramphenicol until the result of bacterial sensitivity testing (if available) is known. Ampicillin may be used in a similar way, or may be used alone if chloramphenicol is not available.

Doses are as follows:

penicillin G   100 000 units/kg per dose
                      intramuscularly or intravenously;
                      3-hourly initially, then 6-hourly when
                      child improves.

ampicillin   100 mg/kg per dose intramuscularly or
                    intravenously; 6-hourly.

Treatment of meningitis should continue for a total of 14
days.

Neonatal meningitis should be treated with penicillin G and
chloramphenicol until CSF culture results are available as
follows.

1. *Term babies up to 1 week of age, and preterm babies up
to 1 month of age:*
penicillin G   50 000 units/kg per dose
                    intramuscularly or intravenously;
                    12-hourly.
chloramphenicol 12.5 mg/kg per dose intramuscularly
                    or intravenously; 12-hourly.
2. *Term babies of more than 1 week and preterm babies of
more than 1 month:*
penicillin G   50 000 units/kg per dose
                    intramuscularly or intravenously;
                    6-hourly.
chloramphenicol 12.5 mg/kg per dose intramuscularly
                    or intravenously; 6-hourly.

Chloramphenicol should not be given orally in the newborn
period. Other drugs sometimes used are ampicillin 50 mg/kg
per dose, 12-hourly in the first week, 6-hourly afterwards,
and gentamycin 2.5 mg/kg per dose 12-hourly in the first
week, 8-hourly afterwards. Treatment should continue for 3
weeks.

Anticonvulsants. Fits should be controlled either with
paraldehyde, 0.2 ml/kg given intramuscularly, or with
diazepam, 0.25 mg/kg given slowly intravenously or 0.5
mg/kg given rectally. These may be repeated in 10 minutes if
there is no effect.

Further fits should be prevented by giving regular

anticonvulsants. Phenobarbitone is given in a loading dose of 15 mg/kg intramuscularly and then a single daily dose of 5 mg/kg. If this is not effective, phenytoin may be given either orally or, preferably, very slowly intravenously in a loading dose of 15 mg/kg and continued orally at 2.5 mg/kg per dose twice daily. Phenytoin should not be given for more than a few days to a child being treated with chloramphenicol. Paraldehyde 0.2 ml/kg per dose diluted 1 in 10 in water may be given 6-hourly by a nasogastric tube, or rectally.

In children who have had fits, anticonvulsants should ideally be continued for up to 1 year after discharge from hospital and then withdrawn slowly, but this is not always possible or practical.

Because of the high incidence of fits occurring in children with meningitis under the age of 2 years, all children in this age group should receive anticonvulsants from the time of admission. If no fits occur, the anticonvulsants can be stopped when the child's general condition is satisfactory.

Antimalarials. In countries where malaria is common, children should receive a treatment course of antimalarials.

Feeding. If the child is not vomiting, and is not feeding, milk (preferably expressed breast milk) should be given by nasogastric tube. It may be necessary to give fluids intravenously in a child who is continuously vomiting, but great care should be taken not to give too much intravenous fluid.

Progress

Most children respond within 24–72 hours to treatment and are visibly improved. It is not necessary to repeat lumbar puncture and cerebrospinal fluid examination unless the child is not improving or, having initially improved, starts to get worse. It is most important, however, to continue treatment with antibiotics for 2 weeks (3 weeks in neonates).

Prevention

Close contacts of patients with meningococcal meningitis should be given a sulphonamide. The dose is 25 mg/kg (maximum 1 g) every 6 hours for 2 days. A meningococcal vaccine is available, and may be useful in epidemic control.

Viral meningitis

Many different viruses can cause meningitis. Mumps virus and enteroviruses (including poliovirus) are two of the most common.

Disease picture

Viral meningitis may occur as part of a more generalized viral illness such as mumps, or measles, or may occur without other associated features. Symptoms and signs are similar to those for bacterial meningitis, but, in general, patients with viral meningitis are less severely ill than those with bacterial meningitis. It is, however, impossible to diagnose viral meningitis on clinical grounds alone, and children suspected of having meningitis must have a lumbar puncture performed for cerebrospinal fluid examination.

Diagnosis

Characteristically, the cerebrospinal fluid contains more lymphocytes than polymorphs. Bacteria are not seen on gram-stain and there is no growth on culture. Protein is often normal, or may be slightly raised, while sugar is usually normal. Unfortunately these findings are not specific for viral meningitis, but may also be found in partly treated bacterial meningitis.

Treatment

If the diagnosis can be made with certainty, treatment with antibiotics is unnecessary. Analgesics are then the only drugs indicated. In practice, however, it is often difficult to decide whether the meningitis is bacterial or viral in origin. In such cases it is safer to treat the child for bacterial meningitis.

Tuberculous meningitis (TBM)

Meningitis due to the tubercle bacillus may occur as part of miliary tuberculosis. More often, however, it arises from the discharge into the cerebrospinal fluid of tubercle bacilli from a focus just below the surface of the brain substance.

Disease picture

The signs and symptoms of TBM are similar to those of bacterial meningitis, but the onset is usually much slower. Frequently, the child has been unwell for several weeks before reaching medical attention.

A history of constipation is common. Occasionally the child may have failed to complete a previous course of TB treatment. On examination, the child usually shows signs of weight loss and there may be lymphadenopathy and abnormal findings in the chest. Neurological abnormalities may be present. A careful family history may reveal affected family members. Occasionally, TB meningitis may present suddenly.

Diagnosis

The cerebrospinal fluid contains an increased number of cells, the majority of which are lymphocytes. Gram-stain shows no organisms. Protein levels are usually raised and are sometimes very high, while the sugar level is low. If left to stand, a gelatinous clot ('pellicle') may appear. Tubercle bacilli may be trapped in the clot and may then be identified by Ziehl–Nielsen staining and microscopic examination. Since few bacilli are present, however, they may easily be missed. Culture results are helpful in confirming the diagnosis, but take 4 to 6 weeks. A chest x-ray may show evidence of miliary TB, or tuberculous bronchopneumonia. Tuberculin tests are usually negative in tuberculous meningitis, but often convert during treatment.

Screening of family contacts with chest x-rays, Mantoux tests and sputum examination may reveal an affected member.

Treatment

Antituberculous drugs.   Treatment regimens vary depending on drug availability and departmental policies. Almost all regimens include streptomycin and isoniazid. Streptomycin is not effective against TB in the meninges or brain, because it does not cross the blood–brain barrier well, and so rifampicin, which does penetrate the cerebrospinal fluid, is usually used as well. Pyrazinamide is also used, particularly in short course treatment regimens.

A satisfactory initial treatment, of 2 to 3 months duration, would be:

streptomycin 30 mg/kg intramuscularly daily
isoniazid 15 mg/kg orally daily
rifampicin 10–15 mg/kg orally daily

Pyrazinamide 30 mg/kg orally daily is added in some short-course regimens. Following initial treatment, treatment with streptomycin and isoniazid (or ethambutol 15 mg/kg and isoniazid) is continued, usually for a total of 12–18 months. Shorter regimens are currently being tested.

Steroids.   Prednisolone should be given in a dose of 2 mg/kg per day in four divided doses for a period of 3 weeks, and then withdrawn gradually.

Anticonvulsants   These may be required.

Feeding   Where the disease is severe, careful attention must be given to the child's nutrition. Nasogastric feeding with a high-calorie and high protein diet supplemented with vitamins and minerals may be required. Expressed breast milk should be given if the child is unable to suck.

Other measures   Good nursing care is most important. If urinary retention occurs, it may be necessary to pass a catheter. Bed-sores must be prevented by frequent turning of the unconscious patient.

Progress

If the TBM is diagnosed and treated early, the outcome is likely to be good. If severe neurological signs are present the outlook is less good, but some severely affected children make a good recovery. Recovery is considerably slower than from bacterial meningitis.

Complications of meningitis

Early complications

Severe cerebral oedema   This usually presents as persistent and uncontrolled fitting, and may be treated by fluid restriction and by the use of dexamethasone in a dose of 0.1 mg/kg 6-hourly or mannitol 1 g/kg intravenously over 1 hour (5 ml/kg 20 per cent mannitol).

Subdural effusion or abscess   This is a collection of fluid beneath the meninges and is a complication of bacterial meningitis. It should be suspected in any child who fails to respond to treatment. Daily measurement will reveal an enlarging head circumference, and the fontanelle will feel full. Such effusions should be drained daily by means of a needle inserted with aseptic technique perpendicularly to the skin surface at the lateral angles of the anterior fontanelle.

Late complications

Hydrocephalus is recognized by finding an abnormally rapid growth of head circumference.

Microcephaly may result from meningitis in babies and infants.

Delayed mental and physical development, persistent paralyses, deafness, and *epilepsy* are common sequelae, usually resulting from late or inadequate treatment. They emphasize the need for a very active approach to the diagnosis and treatment of meningitis.

Encephalitis

Encephalitis is inflammation of the brain substance. It may be caused by a number or organisms, but viruses are most common. Encephalitis may occur in epidemics.

Disease picture

Encephalitis may occur as a separate disease or may complicate other viral illnesses such as measles. The illness may be mild with very few symptoms and signs other than fever and a headache. In the severe form, however, the onset may be both rapid and dramatic. There is a high fever with severe headache and often vomiting. The child may become restless, confused or unconscious, and recurrent fits are a common feature.

Diagnosis

In practical terms, the diagnosis of encephalitis is made by excluding meningitis and other causes of fever and fits such as cerebral malaria. A lumbar puncture should therefore be performed and a blood slide examined for malaria parasites if appropriate (p.117).

Treatment

There is no specific treatment for encephalitis, but anticonvulsants are often required. Temperature reduction with aspirin and cool sponging are important, and good nursing care is essential.

Poliomyelitis

This is an infection of the spinal cord, and sometimes the brain, caused by the poliovirus. This virus is present in the faeces of infected patients. It spreads from person to person by means of faecal contamination (e.g. by unwashed hands) entering the body through the mouth. It multiplies in the intestine and may then spread into the body tissues and eventually into the nervous system.

Disease picture

Infections with poliovirus can be put into two groups.

Non-paralytic poliomyelitis

Unnoticed infection   Most infected patients have no signs or symptoms at all.

Mild infection   The illness usually starts suddenly with fever, sore throat, headache, nausea, loss of appetite and sometimes vomiting and abdominal pain. It may last for a few hours or up to several days.

Major illness   Patients have the same symptoms and signs as those with the minor illness, but they are more severe. They have pain and stiffness of the neck, back and legs, and have the features of viral meningitis (p.154). The illness may last up to 5 days.

Paralytic poliomyelitis

This occurs in only a small number of infected patients. It may start as the mild or severe type of non-paralytic poliomyelitis. Paralysis may follow straight away, or there may be a few days after the early symptoms when the patient seems to be better, before the paralysis occurs. Occasionally, paralysis may occur first. There is often muscle pain before paralysis and usually the amount of paralysis is different on the two sides of the body. In severe cases, the muscles of respiration may be paralysed.

If the brain itself is affected, the centres controlling breathing and swallowing may be damaged. There may be paralysis of the face or eyes.

Diagnosis

Diagnosis is usually made on a clinical basis and is made easier if the disease is occurring commonly, such as in an epidemic. In major non-paralytic and in paralytic poliomyelitis, the cerebrospinal fluid contains an increased number of lymphocytes and has a high protein content.

Treatment

There is no antibiotic treatment for poliomyelitis. *Good mursing care is the most important part of treatment.* Temperature reduction and pain relievers are helpful. Hot soaks or hot baths help to relieve severe muscle pain, and physiotherapy should begin as soon as the pain ceases. Splints may be helpful but should not be applied for long periods of time—since the aim of treatment is to keep paralysed limbs flexible and so prevent contractures. Frequent position changes are important. If the patient has difficulty in breathing and swallowing, artificial ventilation is usually indicated. Antibiotics may be required if chest infection complicates the illness. Intramuscular injections should be avoided in patients with poliomyelitis—since they make paralysis of the injected muscle more likely.

Prevention

Poliomyelitis can be prevented by vaccination with a live vaccine, given by mouth (Sabin), or by inactivated polio virus vaccine given by injection (Salk). Three doses should be given for full vaccination, but epidemics may be controlled by giving all people at risk a single dose of Sabin vaccine.

Tetanus

Tetanus is a disease of the nervous system caused by a chemical substance (exotoxin) produced by the bacteria, *Clostridium tetani*. This organism is excreted in the faeces of many animals and is present in soil and dirt. By producing spores, the organism survives for a long time, and, once it is contaminated, soil remains infective for many years.

The organisms usually enter the body through the site of any injury, which may be very severe or may be so slight that it is not noticed. Infection may enter through the umbilical cord in newborn babies, particularly if the cord is cut with a dirty instrument or is covered with dirt or with dirty dressings. Once inside the body, the bacteria multiply, producing the toxin which affects the nerves, spinal cord and brain.

Disease picture

The most important feature of tetanus is involuntary contractions of muscles (spasms).

In the newborn

Signs and symptoms appear between 3 and 10 days after delivery. The first problem is that the baby cannot suck because of spasm in his jaw muscles. Shortly after this, the baby develops stiffness of the body, and jerking spasms begin. In severe cases, the baby's back may be arched backwards (opisthotonos). An unpleasant strangled type of cry may accompany the spasms.

In children

Symptoms usually begin between 5 and 14 days after the

initial injury, with increasing stiffness of the muscles of the jaw and neck. The jaw may be locked during spasms (trismus or lockjaw) and the patient may appear to be smiling due to spasm of the facial muscles (risus sardonicus). As the disease gets worse, the abdominal wall is affected and the arms and legs also develop spasms. As in babies, arching of the back may occur. Involvement of respiratory muscles and muscles of the larynx and pharynx may lead to death. Urinary retention may occur.

The spasms, which may be started off by noise, bright lights, sudden movement or other more minor stimuli, are painful and exhausting. Frequently, the child is unable to eat or drink. The child may or may not be febrile and usually is fully conscious until the last stages.

Diagnosis

Diagnosis is made on a clinical basis. Care must be taken to distinguish tetanic spasms from convulsions. The arching of the back and neck may resemble the neck stiffness seen in meningitis.

Treatment

Good nursing care

The patient should, if possible, be nursed in a separate, quiet and darkened room, and should be left alone as much as possible. If a separate room is not available, the quietest corner of a busy ward may be screened off. Intramuscular injections should be kept to a minimum. Hydration is maintained initially by intravenous fluids. Subsequently, nutrition may be given via a nasogastric tube (passed after sedation), and this route should be used where possible for administration of sedation.

Sedation

Usually a combination of drugs is required to achieve

adequate sedation. Diazepam and chlorpromazine are extremely useful. To start with, diazepam is given slowly intravenously in a dose of 2 mg/kg, repeated until spasms stop (up to 10 mg/kg). After that, it is given every 6 hours, either intravenously or by nasogastric tube, in a dose of 2–10 mg/kg per dose. Chlorpromazine in a dose of 1–2 mg/kg per dose 6-hourly should be given by nasogastric tube or intramuscularly if necessary. The two drugs are alternated every 3 hours.

Paraldehyde 0.2 ml/kg intramuscularly may be used as an alternative to diazepam for initial sedation, and it may also be used 6-hourly rectally or orally in the same dose (but diluted 1 in 10 in water) for continuous sedation.

If spasms are not controlled by these measures, phenobarbitone 3 mg/kg 6-hourly intravenously may be added. In the most severe cases, it may be necessary to use thiopentone and to paralyse the patient with curare. These measures require the availability of artificial ventilation.

Tetanus immunoglobulin or antitoxin

If the intravenous preparation of human tetanus immuno-globulin is availble a total of 4000 units is given, 250 units intrathecally, the remainder by intravenous infusion. If this is not available give the intramuscular preparation, 750 units on the first day, and 500 units on the next two days (not intra-thecally).

In the absence of human immunoglobulin, tetanus antitoxin 10 000 units is given, half intravenously and half intramuscularly after a test dose.

Cleaning of the wounds

If the wound is still obvious, it should be carefully and thoroughly cleaned. In the newborn, the umbilical stump should be cleaned and antibiotic powder applied.

Antibiotics

A course of penicillin should be given intravenously or orally to kill the tetanus bacilli. If pneumonia develops, it should be treated appropriately.

Immunization

An attack of tetanus does not result in immunity, and a course of immunization with tetanus toxoid should be started when improvement occurs. At least two doses, given 2 months apart, are required.

Prevention

Tetanus is a preventable disease, and immunization with tetanus toxoid is the most important preventive measure. Tetanus immunization, either primary or booster, is an important part of antenatal care. The antibodies produced cross the placenta and protect the newborn baby for the first few months of life. All children should receive a three-dose course of tetanus toxoid, usually given in combination with diphtheria and whooping cough vaccine as 'triple antigen', at 1– to 2–month intervals, starting at 2 to 3 months of age (p.224).

Mothers of affected newborn babies should be immunized during the baby's treatment.

In parts of the world where neonatal tetanus is common, it may be found that the cords are cut with dirty instruments such as an old razor blade or a special 'ceremonial' knife or sharp stone. In some areas it is traditional to 'dress' the cord with cow dung. Health education is obviously vitally important here. In some areas, village midwives–village women with basic training in hygienic methods of delivery and baby care–have greatly reduced the incidence of neonatal tetanus.

In older children, careful cleaning and dressing of wounds is most important.

16
Some infectious diseases

Shanti Ghosh

Whooping cough (pertussis)

This is a highly infectious disease caused by bacteria (*Bordetella pertussis*) and rapidly spreads from one child to another by droplet infection. The disease is highly infectious during the early catarrhal stage, but once the typical spasmodic bouts start, the infectivity becomes negligible. It has a prolonged course of 8–10 weeks, and the local names in various countries reflect its long duration and the peculiar nature of cough. Unlike some other diseases, a newborn baby has no immunity to whooping cough, and can get the disease any time after birth. The disease is very severe in children under the age of 1 year, and most of the deaths due to it occur under that age.

Clinical picture

The incubation period is 1–2 weeks. The disease has a catarrhal and a spasmodic stage. For the first week, the cough is like an ordinary upper respiratory catarrh, but at the end of a week it becomes spasmodic and comes in bouts, initially more often during the night, but later during the day as well. The child goes on coughing, his face becomes red and suffused, the tongue protrudes and the eyes begin to water. At the end of the bout, the child takes a deep breath, and there is a prolonged croaking sound which is called a whoop, which is produced by the air entering through a partially closed glottis (entrance to the larynx). This gives the disease its name. The child brings out sticky secretions from his nose and mouth and very often vomits. At the end of the bout, the child lies back exhausted. In babies, the attacks are atypical. There is a spasm of coughing, the baby stops breathing for a

165

minute or two and becomes cyanosed, then takes a breath and vomits mucus. There is usually no whoop. A longer period without breathing may result in death. In between the attacks of cough, the child looks remarkably well, in contrast to other respiratory infections. The chest examination is usually normal except for some rhonchi.

Gradually, over 3–4 weeks, the bouts of cough and their duration become less and disappear about 8–10 weeks from the beginning of the disease. In immunized children, the disease is mild and atypical.

Diagnosis

During the whooping cough season (late winter and spring), whenever a mother brings a child with cough, history regarding whooping cough in the family or neighbourhood should be elicited. Mothers can usually identify whooping cough as a distinct entity, and will themselves volunteer the information.

The diagnosis is clinical, with a history of typical cough. If available, a blood count usually shows leucocytosis with increased lymphocytes, but in young children the blood count may be normal. During the early catarrhal stage the disease has to be distinguished from other respiratory infections, such as upper respiratory catarrh and bronchitis. The history of contact with whooping cough will help to distinguish it from other conditions. Later, the spasmodic nature of the cough helps in diagnosis.

Treatment

This is entirely symptomatic. Humidification helps to make the secretions less tenacious. To prevent exhaustion and reduce the severity of cough, promethazine in a dose of 1 mg/kg per dose may be given. There is evidence to suggest that in the catarrhal stage, erythromycin 40 mg/kg per day or ampicillin 150 mg/kg per day for about 1 week shortens the duration of illness. Chloramphenicol too may be given in a dose of 50 mg/kg per day if the other drugs are not available. Once the spasmodic stage has set in, antibiotics have no value except in the management of complications.

Complications

Due to the severity of bouts of cough, bleeding can occur into the eyes (under the conjunctiva), from the nose, the lung and, rarely, into the brain, resulting in convulsions. In young children, lung complications such as collapse of a part of the lung are common because of the thick sticky nature of the secretions blocking the passage of air to a part of the lung. Secondary infection may result in pneumonia. There may be convulsions and, rarely, inflammation of the brain. Tuberculosis may become active again due to whooping cough.

Feeding

The prolonged illness and frequent vomiting result in malnutrition, and so every effort should be made to feed the child adequately. Small, frequent semisolid feeds of low bulk and high energy density should be given. Sometimes dry food, like bread or biscuits, provokes a bout of cough. If the child vomits, the feed needs to be repeated.

Isolation

The maximum period of infectivity is the early catarrhal period of 2 weeks, but unless a history of contact is available, it is difficult to diagnose the disease at this stage. Besides, in overcrowded homes, isolation is seldom possible. Every effort should be made to keep infants under 6 months of age away from a suspected case of whooping cough, for 2–3 weeks.

In many countries, it is customary to visit a sick child and take other children along as well. Or a child with whooping cough may be taken along while visiting friends and neighbours. This leads to spread of infection, and is true of all infectious diseases. A better knowledge of spread of infection will gradually help to stop these customs.

Prevention

Whooping cough vaccine should be given as part of DPT (diphtheria, pertussis, tetanus vaccine, p.190). Since there is no acquired immunity through the placenta, the baby should be immunized as soon as possible. Three doses of DPT should be given at 4–6 week intervals, beginning at 2–3 months of age. A booster of DPT should be given at about 2 years. In a field situation, the aim should be to complete the three doses of DPT as early as possible. It may not be possible to give more than two doses.

Measles

Measles is a highly infectious disease caused by a virus, and spreads by droplet infection from one child to another through coughing, sneezing or talking. There are several taboos regarding measles in most countries. In India, it can be considered a visitation by a goddess, and thus to be left alone. Because of overcrowding, infection spreads rapidly among the children. In most developing countries, most children have had measles before the age of 3–4 years. The disease confers a life-long immunity, and the baby has some immunity for the first 6 months of life because of the immunity acquired through the placenta. The immunity wanes rapidly after that, and by 1 year of age, one-third of children will have suffered from the disease, and by 3 years three-quarters will have suffered from it. This has relevance to the timing of measles immunization.

Clinical picture

The incubation period is 10–12 days. The disease starts with cough, a running nose and fever and, unless the history of contact is available, it may be passed off as an upper respiratory infection. This is the stage when the disease is highly infectious. With experience, this stage can be distinguished from an ordinary cold—the face looks suffused, there is watering of the eyes and the eyelids are puffy. The mouth should be examined for Koplik' spots, which are small, whitish lesions like grains of salt on the cheeks, particularly near the lower molars, and are characteristic of measles. After 3–4 days, a fine macular rash develops along the hair line and the posterior part of the cheeks. The rash becomes maculopapular, and gradually spreads to the rest of the body during the next day or two, and this is the period of maximum coryza, cough and fever. Once the rash reaches the legs, it begins to disappear from the face. About a week later, skin begins to peel off (desquamation) and there is pigmentation of the skin, which may last for weeks. In severe measles, the rash is darker and runs together into large patches, and there is much more desquamation. The rash may even be haemorrhagic in severe disease. Fever and cough gradually subside as the rash fades. If fever continues to be high, and the cough persists, some chest complication should be suspected. The disease is severe in malnourished and young children, and leads to further malnutrition, resulting in marasmus or kwashiorkor. Deaths mainly occur in young malnourished children. The incidence varies in different studies, but it is now generally agreed that the disease is severe enough to warrant immunization, and measles immunization now forms a part of the Expanded Programme of Immunization in almost all countries.

Complications

Common complications include conjunctivitis, otitis media, stomatitis, laryngitis, bronchitis, pneumonia and diarrhoea. There may be ulceration of the skin. Cancrum oris (gangrenous infection of the mouth) may develop in malnourished children. In malnourished children, particularly those with vitamin A deficiency, conjunctivitis may lead to blindness. If fever and cough do not subside with the disappearance of the rash, some chest complication should be suspected. Primary tuberculous lesion may flare up following measles due to lowered resistance. Rarely, the disease may lead to encephalitis. The child may become semiconscious or comatose, and there may be convulsions.

Treatment

This is mainly symptomatic, and consists of medicines for fever (usually aspirin) and soothing lotion for the skin. During the height of the rash, cool sponging of the whole body will help to bring down the temperature. Overclothing in the belief that it helps to 'bring out' the rash should be avoided, as it may lead to seriously high temperatures (hyperpyrexia). The irritating cough will respond to promethazine 1 mg/kg dose. The eyes should be washed frequently with clean water. If there is conjunctivitis, antibiotic drops or ointments may be necessary. Antibiotics play no role in the treatment of uncomplicated measles. If pneumonia or other respiratory infections occur, then antibiotics will have to be used. Penicillin, erythromycin or ampicillin may be used in appropriate dosage. Severe diarrhoea may result in dehydration, and so care should be taken to advise adequate fluids by mouth.

Nutrition

As mentioned earlier, measles leads to worsening of the nutritional status of the child. During the height of illness, the child is ill and toxic, and has poor appetite. Sometimes food may be withheld due to ignorance and prejudice. Soreness of the mouth too prevents the child from eating. Diarrhoea causes less absorption of food. Every effort should be made to coax the child to eat as much as possible. Small, frequent, high-energy density feeds should be given.

Isolation

It is not possible to observe isolation in a crowded household. Maximum period of infectivity is the catarrhal phase before the rash develops and before the diagnosis is confirmed, and so attempts at isolation once the disease is diagnosed are no use and do not prevent the spread of infection.

Prevention

Measles vaccine confers a prolonged immunity, probably life long. Keeping in view the age incidence of measles in developing countries, the most suitable time for immunization is around 9 months.

Typhoid

Typhoid fever is common in countries where standards of personal hygiene and sanitation are poor. It is caused by bacteria (*Salmonella typhi.*) The infected persons excrete the bacilli in the stool and urine. Infection is caused by eating infected food or drinking infected water or milk. Food and water may be contaminated by the hands of the carriers, or through flies. The small intestines develop ulcers and the bacteria enter the bloodstream. Infectivity lasts as long as the bacteria are present in stool or urine. A few patients continue to excrete bacteria in their stool and are called 'carriers'. These people are an important source of spread of infection, particularly if they happen to be food handlers. The carrier state is uncommon in children.

Clinical picture

The incubation period is about 14 days. The disease most commonly affects schoolchildren and is uncommon under 2 years of age. The severity of the disease varies a great deal, and is no less severe in children compared with adults. In young children, the presentation is variable and atypical. The onset is gradual and the temperature rises gradually for 1 week. A maculopapular rash (rose spots) may be seen on the chest and abdomen, but is difficult to see on dark skin. Sometimes the onset may be sudden, with headache, cough, vomiting and diarrhoea. Even though typically the fever is of a continuous type, intermittent fever is also not uncommon. The child looks ill and toxic, the tongue is coated, there may be abdominal pain with some distension. Diarrhoea is present in almost half the patients. The commonly described slow pulse in relation to the fever in adults is usually not seen in children. Bronchitis is common. Sometimes the patient may become delirious or drowsy in the second week (typhoid state). The spleen is palpable 2–3 cm below the costal margin and is soft. The liver, too, may become enlarged and there may be mild jaundice. Chest examination shows signs of bronchitis, and sometimes pneumonia. Fever lasts for about 3 weeks and comes down gradually. With the use of antibiotics, fever comes down earlier. Relapse may occur in 5–10 per cent of cases and the usual time is about 2 weeks after fever has come down. Relapse is usually milder than the original illness.

Diagnosis

In the initial stage, the disease may resemble influenza, bronchitis or gastroenteritis. However, fever for more than 1 week, with distension of the abdomen and a palpable spleen, suggests typhoid. The blood count may show reduced white blood cells. A positive blood culture (finding of typhoid bacilli in blood) confirms the diagnosis. A serological test (Widal test) is not diagnostic, even though high titres are suggestive.

Complications

There may be severe watery diarrhoea, pneumonia, or encephalopathy. Intestinal haemorrhage and perforation are severe complications. There is usually a rapid pulse, abdominal pain and distension, preceding these complications. Later, there is pallor and shock. Following perforation, peritonitis develops, and the abdomen becomes rigid.

Treatment

Bedrest is essential while there is fever. The diet should be high in protein and calories. There are often many prejudices and beliefs regarding diet in typhoid. It may be believed that any solid, particularly cereal grain, foods are harmful. This is not so, and anything the child fancies can be given. Often the child has to be coaxed to eat because of poor appetite.

Cool sponging may bring down the temperature. Diarrhoea may result in dehydration, and adequate fluids should be given by mouth and, if necessary, intravenously.

Chloramphenicol in a dose of 50 mg/kg per day is the drug of choice. The drug is usually given for 7 days after fever has subsided. Some authorities advise the administration of the drug for a total period of 3 weeks. Ampicillin (100–200 mg/kg per day) may also be given. It is less effective than chloramphenicol, but is better for preventing a relapse.

Prevention

Improvement of environmental hygiene and sanitation, discouraging fly breeding, and adequate quantities of a safe water supply are essential for prevention of the disease. Latrines should be provided and people should be encouraged to use them for passing both stools and urine.

Water should be taken from either a municipal system or a deep well. It should be stored in covered pots, and a long-handled ladle should be used for taking it out. If the source of drinking water is unsafe, it can be purified by boiling for 5–10 minutes after straining through a clean cloth, or by adding bleaching powder, 20 mg to 1 gallon (about 5 litres) of water. Exposed food from roadside stalls should not be eaten. Patients with typhoid can be nursed in open wards, but their urine and stools should be treated with caution—they should be soaked for 2–3 hours in a 1 : 20 solution of carbolic acid before being poured into a sluice or a pit latrine. Clothes and bed-linen should be similarly treated before being washed. Strict handwashing is essential after every visit to the patient. Flies should be eliminated to the extent possible. Hands should be washed before eating or serving food.

Typhoid vaccine has been shown to be effective for 3–4 years in a majority of cases. Acetone-inactivated vaccine is better than a heat-phenol-inactivated vaccine. Two injections should be given subcutaneously at an interval of 4 weeks. The vaccine can be given intradermally also. Typhoid immunization can be included in the immunization schedule of children, starting at about 3–4 years of age. It can be given at school entry age if it has not already been given. Currently, however, most immunization programmes correctly give emphasis to more common childhood infections (e.g. whooping cough, measles, poliomyelitis etc., p. 190).

Recently, an oral typhoid vaccine, Ty 21a, has been developed and found to be highly effective in field trials. The vaccine is stable and safe, and is highly protective for at least 3 years. However, the vaccine is not yet available for general use.

Leprosy

Leprosy is a chronic communicable disease caused by the leprosy bacillus (*Mycobacterium leprae*), which enters the body through the skin or nose. The skin and nerves are most involved. In endemic countries, the infection occurs mainly during childhood. The disease is uncommonly recognized before the age of 5 years, and is mostly seen in children in the age group 5–14 years. Infection is acquired from infected parents or from some other member of the family, but sometimes the source of infection cannot be traced.

Method of transmission

The bacilli are discharged from ulcers in the nose, throat or skin, and enter the body through small injuries or ulcerations in the skin, or even through normal-looking skin. The bacilli may enter the body through the upper respiratory tract. There is some evidence that bites of mosquitoes and bedbugs may also transmit disease. Infection depends on the infectivity of the leprosy case and the susceptibility of the exposed person. Fortunately, not all cases are infectious. Infectivity can be determined by examining the skin scrapings and nose smears for leprosy bacilli.

Clinical picture

The incubation period varies from a few months to several years, but is commonly between 2 and 5 years.

The most common sign in children is a patch in the skin (macule) which is lighter in colour than the surrounding skin, and in which there is loss of feeling to touch, temperature and pain.

Thickening of skin on the face and hands can occur, which becomes red and shiny. In some cases, loss of feeling, numbness, or a feeling of pins and needles in hands and feet can develop. The nerves most involved are those of the arm, the face and behind the ears. They become thickened and can be easily felt and even seen. Deformities, ulcers and loss of fingers and toes are very rarely seen in children.

Diagnosis

The diagnosis of leprosy can be established in most children by clinical examination only, i.e. finding of a patch on the skin, loss of sensation in the patch, and thickening of nerves. Nose swab and scrapings from the skin should be examined for leprosy bacilli.

Treatment

Even though leprosy can have a spontaneous cure, it is not possible to predict the outcome in any case. So all cases have to be treated. The treatment should be started as soon as the diagnosis is made, with dapsone (DDS, diaminodiphenyl sulphone) tablets. The drug is cheap. The treatment should be continued until all signs of activity of the disease subside, and for 2 to 3 years after that. Treatment is best given for 6 days in a week, the seventh one being a rest day. It can also be given once a week, but is less satisfactory, even though much more convenient from the patient's point of view. A smaller dose should be given to start with, and the maximum dose should be reached in 6–8 weeks.

Another schedule of treatment is to give a quarter of the total weekly dosage in the first month, one-half during the second month, three-quarters in the third month, and the full dosage in the fourth month. Treatment should be maintained at the same dosage. Irregular treatment may lead to drug resistance; improvement stops, and the clinical condition begins to deteriorate.

To prevent the emergence of secondary sulphone resistance, a WHO Expert Committee has recommended that combined treatment should be given initially to lepromatous and borderline cases. As well as full dosage of sulphone, clofazimine (Lamprene) at a dosage of 100 mg daily or 100 mg three times a week should be given for the first 4–6 weeks of treatment. After that, sulphone should be continued. Another regimen suggested by the Expert Committee is sulphone combined with rifampicin at the dosage of 300-600 mg daily for a minimum of 2 weeks. The cost of these drugs is high, and that poses a major problem.

Prognosis

The prognosis in children treated early and adequately is excellent.

Prevention

Vaccination with BCG gives some protection against leprosy. Dapsone in small doses has been shown to have a protective value. This is given twice a week in a dose of 10 mg between the ages of 0 and 2 years, 25 mg between 3 and 5 years, and 50 mg between 6 and 10 years. If a mother is under regular DDS therapy, there is no need for prophylaxis in a breast-fed baby because the baby will get adequate amounts of DDS from breast milk. The duration of prophylactic treatment should be for 3 years after the source case becomes non-infective, or is removed from contact with the child.

In an endemic area, regular screening of schoolchildren for any signs of leprosy should be carried out. The whole body should be examined in a good light.

Education of public

There is a great deal of ignorance about leprosy, and it is considered a social stigma. This may delay diagnosis and treatment because of the resistance concerning examination and diagnosis. There is a great need for health education of the children suffering from leprosy and their families, school health authorities, school teachers, all health personnel and the community. There is no need to isolate the child, and he can continue to attend school.

Diphtheria

This is an acute infectious disease caused by the bacteria *Corynebacterium diphtheriae*. It is acquired by contact with either a carrier or a person with the disease. Disease spreads by droplet infection by coughing, sneezing or talking. The maximum incidence is in spring and autumn. A baby has immunity for the first 4–6 months of life.

Clinical picture

The incubation period is 1–6 days. There is low-grade fever, a general feeling of being unwell (malaise), and aches and pains. The child looks more ill than would be expected with the low fever. Symptoms vary with the site of the disease.

Nasal diphtheria

This resembles a common cold, the discharge gradually becoming mucopurulent with a foul odour. There is excoriation (sores) of the nostrils and upper lip. This form of disease is relatively mild and occurs mostly in infants.

Tonsillar and pharyngeal diphtheria

This form of disease is more severe. There is very poor appetite, malaise, headache, fever and sore throat, and the child looks ill and toxic. After 1–2 days, a greyish membrane forms on the tonsils, and may spread beyond the tonsils to the palate or to pharynx. Removal of the membrane results in bleeding. There is a foul smell from the mouth. Glands in the neck enlarge and sometimes resemble bull-neck. The membrane peels off in 7–10 days.

Laryngeal diphtheria

There is noisy breathing, stridor, hoarseness and dry cough. There is difficulty in breathing with sucking in above the clavicles and beneath the ribs (suprasternal and subcostal retraction). Later, there is cyanosis, and death occurs due to inability to breathe enough air unless the obstruction is relieved.

Diagnosis

This is clinical. Culture of a throat swab will confirm the diagnosis, but treatment should be started as soon as a clinical diagnosis has been made. In the nasal form, the disease has to be differentiated from a cold, or from a foreign body (such as a peanut) pushed up the nose by the child. The tonsillar form may be mistaken for tonsillitis. However, in tonsillitis, fever is high, the child is not particularly toxic, and the membrane is whitish and limited to the tonsils. The laryngeal form should be differentiated from tracheolaryngitis and from a foreign body in the air passages.

Complications

Involvement of heart muscle (myocarditis) is a serious complication and may lead to death. Nerve paralysis can also occur. There may be paralysis of the soft palate, usually in the third week, resulting in difficulty in swallowing, a nasal voice and regurgitation of fluids through the nose. Involvement of nerves of the eye leads to blurring of vision, difficulty in focusing and squint. Other nerves may also be involved, leading to weakness and paralysis.

Treatment

Complete recovery occurs in a few weeks. Complete rest in bed is essential to prevent heart complications. Aspirin should be given to relieve fever and headache. Care should be taken to give adequate fluids and diet. Procaine pencillin 600 000 units a day, or erythromycin 40 mg/kg per day, should be given for 7–10 days. Treatment should be continued until three consecutive throat swabs are negative for diphtheria bacilli.

Diphtheria antitoxin should be given as soon as possible. The dose varies from 40 000 to 80 000 units, depending on the severity and the site of the disease. A sensitivity test should be carried out before administering the antitoxin; 0.1 ml of 1 : 1000 dilution of antitoxin is injected intracutaneously. In a sensitive case, there will be an erythema of 10 mm or more within 20 minutes. In the case of a positive sensitivity test, desensitization is undertaken.

The remaining antitoxin should be given intravenously, slowly. Epinephrine 1 in 1000 solution should be kept ready in a syringe and administered intravenously in the case of a reaction.

Laryngeal obstruction may require tracheostomy (opening an airway into the trachea), and should not be delayed until the child becomes cyanosed or goes into shock.

Prevention

A case of diphtheria should be isolated until all signs of the disease have disappeared, and three consecutive throat swabs are negative for diphtheria bacilli. If possible, contacts should have their throat swabs examined, and should be given procaine penicillin 600 000 units daily for 4 days. Erythromycin may also be given instead of penicillin.

Immunization

Three doses of DPT at 4–6 weeks intervals should be given to all children as early as possible—preferably beginning around 2–3 months of age. A booster is given at 1½–2 years, and DT (diphtheria and tetanus toxoid) at school entry.

17
Diseases of the eyes

Hafiz el Shizali

Congenital cataracts

These are relatively common. They usually affect both eyes. The commonest causes are genetic (inherited), or maternal infection with rubella (German measles) during pregnancy. The opacities of the lenses vary in density. Other congenital abnormalities of the eye are frequently present. For treatment, the infant should be sent to an eye specialist, if possible, as a simple operation may be curative.

Inflammatory diseases

Conjunctivitis is very common. In some regions, gonococcal infection is on the increase again. It occurs at birth if the mother has gonococcal infection of the birth canal. The infant's eyes are red, smaller, and there is purulent discharge. Antenatal treatment of the mother and prophylactic penicillin eye-drops given to the baby at birth (p.27) will reduce the incidence. Infected neonates should receive antibiotics locally and intramuscularly. Other bacteria can also cause acute conjunctivitis.

Trachoma virus is the commonest cause of chronic conjunctivitis. It occurs particularly in dry, dusty regions where hygiene is poor and malnutrition common. Infection is spread by close family contact and flies. In the early stages of the infection, the eyes are sore and watery and the inner surface of the eyelids shows the presence of numerous little red, raised spots (follicles). Treatment is with sulphacetamide drops (10–30 per cent solution) and tetracycline ointment. Oral long-acting sulphonamides also help. Later, healing occurs, but may produce scarring of the upper eyelids. This pulls the eyelashes down until they rub on the cornea, leading to blindness. Treatment then is surgical plus antibiotics.

Prevention is by cleanliness, better diet, control of flies, and mass surveys for early detection and treatment.

Nutritional

Vitamin A deficiency (p.96) is the commonest cause of blindness in many tropical countries. It affects mainly young children, especially those with protein-energy malnutrition (p.65). The most serious form is when the cornea becomes dry, cloudy and wrinkled (keratomalacia), as it may eventually burst. Blindness is due to destruction and infection of the eye, or residual scarring of the cornea. Treatment should be started as early as possible by giving vitamin A, 100 000 units intramuscularly, plus antibiotics.

Prevention can be attempted by giving pregnant and lactating mothers and infants a diet rich in carotene (p.97). In areas where vitamin A deficiency is common, large doses of vitamin A can be given intramuscularly every 6 months.

Trauma

Traumatic injuries to the eye are another common cause of blindness. The injury might be due to a foreign body (dust, a piece of metal), a chemical (caustics), sharp instruments, finger-nails of babies, or a direct blow to the eye. All children with such a history or with pain in the eye should have their eyes carefully examined. Fluorescein eye-drops can be useful in showing the size and position of an ulcer. Atropine eye-drops and antibiotic eye ointment, together with a pad and bandage, may be needed. The child should be referred to an eye specialist, if possible.

18
Skin diseases

Erasmus Harland

The heat and humidity in many tropical countries, together with a lack of water for washing, increase the risk of secondary infection of minor skin conditions. Crowded housing increases the risk of spread of skin infections.

Scabies

The typical picture consists of raised, itchy burrows between the fingers and on the wrists and elbows, in which the adult female mite is found. However, red, raised spots occur on other parts of the body, producing severe itching in the groin, genital area, trunk and hands which is worse at night. Secondary bacterial infection may lead to impetigo, often on the buttocks, legs, feet and hands.

Treatment consists of a hot bath of the whole body, the application of benzyl benzoate (25 per cent) or gamma benzene hexachloride (1 per cent) over the whole body, and a repeat bath after 24 hours. If impetigo is present, it should be treated (see below).

Spread is usually by close contact with an infected person. Prevention consists of encouraging daily washing of the whole body and washing all clothing and bedding and leaving them in the sun. All family members should be treated.

Impetigo

This can occur by itself or following secondary infection of scabies. It is a skin infection with streptococci. The infection commences as areas of redness followed by small vesicles (blisters), which then burst and leave circular, oozing, crusted tops.

The condition is very contagious (spreading by contact). In

some cases, the streptococcus infection can lead to kidney disease.

Local antibiotic cream, such as 'Fucidin', should be applied after the crusts have been removed with antiseptic soap such as 'Cetavlon'. If nothing else is available, gentian violet solution (2 per cent) should be used. In severe cases, antibiotics, preferably long acting, for example penicillin or others, should be given.'

Prevention is mainly by cleanliness, which is often restricted by a limited water supply. Personal hygiene and handwashing by health staff between patients prevent spread of the infection.

Bullous impetigo

Large fluid-containing blisters (bullae) may follow infection of the skin with staphylococci. This is especially likely to occur in the newborn. Intramuscular penicillin (or other appropriate antibiotics should be used, as spread to the bloodstream (septicaemia) is likely.

Boils

These usually result from staphylococcal infection of hair follicles. They respond to penicillin or other antibiotics or, if fully developed, to incision and drainage.

Prickly heat

This condition is most common in obese, overdressed babies. It occurs as an itchy rash made up of raised, red spots (papules). Secondary infection can occur, or scratching can lead to red, raw, weeping areas in the moist parts of the neck, groin or axillae. It is caused by swelling and blockage of the sweat glands, which then may become infected. It occurs more readily following excessive washing with soap.

Treatment consists of avoidance of both soap and water for 7 days, keeping affected parts dry with dusting powder, and keeping babies naked and in a draught when the weather is excessively hot and humid.

Diaper dermatitis

In most tropical areas, this problem does not occur, as diapers (nappies) are not used. In more urbanised areas, the condition occurs in babies with infrequently or improperly washed diapers. A raw, red rash around the groin and buttock area is seen, often complicated by vesicles (blisters) or pustules (pus-filled blisters), indicating secondary bacterial infection, or a distinct raised edge suggesting fungus infection. In such cases, fungus infection (thrush) should be looked for in the mouth and, if present, treated with nystatin or gentian violet paint.

Treatment includes attention to the cleanliness of the diapers used, exposure to the air, and the use of nystatin, antibiotic or steroid cream, as indicated.

Prevention is by thoroughly rinsing diapers after washing, by avoiding the use of plastic diaper covers, and by keeping the baby naked as much as possible.

Fungal infections

Small circular areas of light coloured skin (depigmentation) seen on the trunk or shoulders are usually due to infection with the fungus *tinea versicolor*. Treatment consists of a daily bath and application of 2.5 per cent selenium sulphide once daily.

Larger, circular, scaly areas on the scalp, associated with loss of hair, are due to various forms of ringworm of the scalp. Treatment can be given using Whitfield's ointment (salicylic and benzoic acids), or by giving griseofulvin by mouth, especially if the nails are involved.

Cutaneous larva migrans

'Creeping eruption' caused by the larva of *Ancylostoma*

braziliense or *A. caninum* follows infection of the skin with the larvae of a dog hookworm. This irritating rash moves slowly through the skin, leaving an irregular track.

Treatment can be given by applying thiabendazole ointment. Prevention depends on keeping the areas where children play free from defaecating dogs.

Atopic eczema (infantile eczema)

This allergic condition is especially common in infants fed cow's milk in early infancy. It consists of a red, scaly, thickened rash. It often occurs in the flexures (behind the knees, in the arm pits, in front of the elbows), often affecting both sides of the body at the same time. It can also occur on the cheeks. Itching is the main symptom and the resulting scratching may lead to secondary bacterial infection. When present on the scalp, it may lead to 'cradle cap', a matted crust developing over the whole scalp.

Treatment consists of removing the cause of the allergy, using emulsifying cream, applying 1 per cent hydrocortisone cream, and restricting the use of soap and water.

Prevention can be undertaken by breast-feeding *alone* for at least 4 months. Restriction of the mother's intake of cow's milk may be helpful, especially in babies of parents with allergic conditions.

19
Accidents

Mahmoud Mohamed Hassan

Accidents are common in children, particularly under the age of 5 years, owing to the inquisitive nature at this stage of their development. Accidents usually occur at times when nobody is supervising the activities of the child, especially when the mother is absent or sick. The frequency is increased in broken homes, and among children whose vision, hearing or intelligence is impaired or who suffer from epilepsy or physical handicap. Rehabilitation using low-cost, appropriate technology should be part of primary health care services.

Types of accidents, treatment and prevention

1. *Burns and scalds* carry a high risk of mortality in children, especially those in poor homes and overcrowded environments. Those who survive may suffer from disfigurement and psychological trauma, as a result of a painful and prolonged stay in hospital. The most common cause is scalding by hot water, tea or soup when the toddler pulls a hot pot from a stove. Burning of clothes is particularly dangerous. In certain tropical areas, house fires are common in dry seasons and may lead to tragic results.

Treatment of burns should be done in hospital. Shock and respiratory involvement, especially in cases of exposure to smoke, is a serious emergency in certain cases, and requires urgent management. The extent and depth of burn should be evaluated. There is urgent need for prevention of infection, protection of skin, and treatment of anaemia and loss of protein (hypoproteinaemia). After recovery, physiotherapy and rehabilitation may be required.

Burns are preventable by proper care and health education. Safe stoves should be constructed. Methods to prevent children from entering kitchens, especially during the time of cooking, should be adopted.

187

2. *Drowning* may be a common cause of mortality in children, especially those who dwell near rivers and lakes. Prevention depends on adequate parental supervision and on teaching children how to swim from an early age. Early resuscitative measures are vital for saving lives.

3. The incidence of *road accidents* is rising steeply in developing countries, with improvements in roads and increase in number of vehicles. It is advisable to introduce programmes of traffic education to children at schools as early as possible. Young cyclists should learn about safety measures on roads. The use of car seat belts by both adults and children is recommended.

4. *Injuries due to falls* at home and in play grounds may cause fractures, haemorrhage or other complications,and they need proper assessment and treatment. *Bites* by dogs are particularly important where rabies is endemic. The incidence of *electric shock* is increasing in the tropics, especially in big towns, and great care in the installation of wires far from the reach of children is needed.

5. *Poisoning*: accidental poisoning is common in homes where proper care is lacking. Three types of substances may be ingested by children.

(a) *Drugs*, usually prescribed for adults and which are carelessly left within the reach of children. The commonest drugs are: salicylates, iron, barbiturates, anti-histamines, anti-depressants, chloroquine, pyrimethamine (Daraprim).

(b) *Household substances and garden products*: e.g. kerosene, alcohol, insecticides, DDT solutions, caustic soda, disinfectants, paraffin, petrol, phenols.

(c) *Poisonous berries*, plants, seeds and roots, which vary in type according to the specific environment.

Principles of management in poisoning

1. Inquiry and inspection of poison for its identification.
2. Producing vomiting using syrup of ipecacuanha 15 ml

followed by copious drinks of water. It is contraindicated in cases of coma or convulsions and in children who have swallowed caustic substances (strong acids, strong alkalis, phenols) and hydrocarbons (kerosene, paraffin, petrol).

3. Stomach washout is needed in the case of most swallowed poisons. The stomach is washed as soon as possible with several pints of plain water. Gastric contents should be kept and sent for laboratory investigations if possible. Gastric lavage is contraindicated in cases of kerosene and caustics. In cases of iron poisoning, sodium bicarbonate solution is used for gastric lavage and a small amount is left in the stomach.

4. Acids and alkalis are diluted by drinking milk or water.

5. Shocked or collapsed children need urgent resuscitation in hospital.

6. Kerosene poisoning may cause chemical aspiration pneumonia and a broad-spectrum antibiotic, e.g. ampicillin, is used to minimize secondary bacterial infection.

Prevention

Accidental poisoning in children can be prevented by keeping drugs locked in cupboards before and after use. Household and other poisonous substances should be kept in stores away from the hands of children. Health education through all available media will enlighten parents to possible unforeseen risks to their children.

20
Health education

E.F. Patrice Jelliffe

Young children and their mothers are often called an 'at-risk' group, as they frequently develop health problems which could be prevented if the parents of the children and the mothers themselves knew and understood the causes of diseases and ways to avoid becoming ill.

Health education, which includes nutrition guidance, may be required for all people in the community. This may include the family unit, i.e. both parents, the older brothers and sisters of the sick child, and all other relatives, so they may help each other to keep well.

Prevention of ill-health

Both simple and cheap ways, as well as expensive and elaborate methods, exist, but none of these will be effective unless individuals in the community can make use of the help given to them in the way it was intended. For example, if a good water supply and latrines are provided by the government to all families in a village in which the majority of children suffer from diarrhoea for many months of the year, and most of the population is infected with roundworms and hookworms, very little benefit will result if the villagers continue to defaecate on the ground around their houses and use the latrine as a small storage unit, and if they do not wash their hands after defaecation and before preparing meals. Any health education which may have been given when these improvements in environmental sanitation were made was an obvious failure, as the relationship between flies, dirty hands, food contamination and diarrhoea, as well as faecal contamination of the soil with ova and larvae of parasites and transmission of disease, was not understood. The villagers had acquired little or no knowledge, had not changed their

190

attitude and, more importantly, their behaviour. Possibly, the health educator had not looked for possible 'cultural blocks' (p.15), which may have prevented them from following the advice, or may have had few 'communication skills'.

What is meant by health education?

Health education implies that people from many disciplines, such as medicine, public health, nutrition, agriculture, etc., who have a good grasp of their subject and know how to teach, can effectively put over a scientifically correct and culturally appropriate message in a very practical way to others in need of help who have little or no modern knowledge of the subject, but who have a long experience in living in the area and much local wisdom.

However, it is easier to provide knowledge than to change attitudes and behaviour. Most people will only alter old habits if they recognize some real benefits for themselves and their families. For example, they may see that neighbours in the community who follow the advice of a nurse and a public health inspector have fewer episodes of illness, can work longer hours, make more money, and are improving their homes etc. These may encourage other families to do the same.

Why should health and nutrition education by taught together?

It is difficult to separate one subject from the other, as they are so closely linked. A child weakened by malaria will be more likely to become malnourished because of high fever, loss of appetite, diarrhoea, etc. Malnutrition, on the other hand, makes a child more susceptible to severe viral or bacterial diseases because of a low resistance to infections (p.67).

Who can teach health education?

In the past, most health education was given by health professionals, as well as by nutritionists, dietitians, home inspectors and nurses, health visitors, medical assistants, etc.). Nutrition education was undertaken in part by health professional, as well as by nutritionists, dietitians, home economists, and some dentists and extension officers in comunity development and agriculture. In recent years, with the idea of 'primary health care',* it has been realized that many other groups should be involved, who, if given basic training, could extend the network of communication on prevention very greatly. These include, among others, teachers, community leaders and volunteers, village midwives, and mothers themselves. The message given by these groups must be the same to avoid confusion in the people's minds, and should not conflict with government policies and programmes in the prevention of malnutrition and disease.

What subjects should the health educator know about?

These will vary with the training of the educator. A physician may have more knowledge for teaching about infectious disease transmission and immunizations (provided he does not overcomplicate) than a village mother, who herself is very well able to teach other mothers how to weigh their babies or make a nutritious 'multimix' (p.61).

However, different types of information are necessary before commencing a health education programme. The following are some examples.

---

* *Primary health care* is essential health care based on practical, scientifically sound and socially acceptable methods and technology, made universally accessible to individuals and families in the community through their full participation, at a cost that the community and country can afford to maintain at every stage of their development in the spirit of self-reliance and self-determination (World Health Organization, Geneva 1978).

1. *The community situation.* For example, the community's needs in terms of nutrition and health, the general economic level, their education (whether they can read and write or are illiterate), as well as their cultural belief about food and illnesses. Details about the treatment they choose (use of charms, herbal medicines, etc.) to aid them when they are sick, and the types of practitioners they will consult, e.g. herbalists, bone setters, etc., and whether they attend government health clinics, if these are available within reasonable distance from their homes. The situation regarding environmental sanitation (water, excreta disposal) should be known.

2. *The important infections in the community.* Some such infections may be constantly present (endemic), such as malaria (p.117) or schistosomiasis (p.115); others occur at certain seasons or in epidemics, such as poliomyelitis (p.159), diphtheria (p.177), measles (p.168) and whooping cough (p.165).

3. *Main nutritional deficiencies.* The main forms of malnutrition need to be known, including the age-groups affected and details of causation. These include different forms of protein-energy malnutrition (PEM), vitamin A deficiency, iron deficiency etc.

4. *Foods grown year round and seasonally*: particularly the staple, the main legumes and 'animal products' (p.61).

5. *Foods sold in the market place or in stores*: their availability, cost, and nutrient value.

6. *Methods of preparing foods*: the popular recipes, especially those used for infant and maternal feeding, the type of fuel and cooking stoves used, as well as cooking vessels and measures employed.

Without this, and similar information, the health educator will not be able to prepare a suitable programme to meet both the 'felt needs' of the community and the actual health needs, nor to communicate appropriately with the people attending the classes or those talking to the educator in clinics or in their homes.

Which topics should be included?

The emphasis must be placed on the most important problems which exist in the community, and those which are recognized as problems by the community. These will vary from one region of a country to another. In most developing countries, a general pattern is seen, and suitable topics would include the following. (1) *General health care*: 7 out of every 10 children born in the poorer parts of the world are never seen by a health worker, so that information on the availability of services is important. (2) *Nutrition*: at least 1 child out of 3 is inadequately nourished and, therefore, in poor health. (3) *Water and sanitation*: 4 out of every 5 children in rural areas of the Third World do not have an adequate water supply or safe sanitation.

Health care

1. The use of maternal and child health care centres (p.215).

2. The need for immunization of children (p.201) against major infectious diseases and of mothers against tetanus.

3. Prevention of diarrhoea (p.102) and worm infections (p.110).

4. Learning simple home remedies including oral rehydration (p.106) of children or adults with diarrhoea.

5. Prevention of accidents in the home (p.187), especially poisoning (e.g. kerosene), burns, scalds and cuts, and their first-aid treatment.

6. Learning when to bring a sick person into the hospital, i.e. recognizing that a child is malnourished, understanding the meaning of weight charts (p.227), recognizing 'night blindness' (p.97), etc.

7. Understanding the method of spread of major infections (e.g. malaria, p.117, schistosomiasis, p.115, etc.), how to prevent their spread (i.e. by killing mosquito larvae, keeping water receptacles covered, not bathing in contaminated rivers or streams, etc.), and other common diseases (e.g. tuber-

culosis, p.135, tetanus of the newborn, p.37, eye diseases, p.181, etc.).

Nutrition

1. Maternal feeding in pregnancy and lactation (p.6).

2. Young child feeding (p.52), breast-feeding, artificial feeding (only when really necessary), introduction of suitable semi solids (multimixes) using culturally acceptable, preferably home-grown, foods.

3. Methods of family spacing (p.217) suitable to the individual family.

4. Nutrition of schoolchildren (p.238) — packed lunches, dental health etc.

5. Food availability, home grown or purchased (best buys for money).

6. Food preservation and processing at home level, improved granaries, prevention of food losses, drying, salting, pickling of foods.

7. Use of simple technology—paddy huskers, manioc graters etc.

As women are often in charge not only of the health of the families, but also of growing, processing and preserving food, it is important that, when possible, they should be helped to lighten their heavy workload by learning about available, new, simple, low-cost methods which have been developed (e.g. ways of grinding, village stores, etc.).

Water and sanitation

1. The availability and use of safe water; use of simple filtering devices.

2. Cleanliness of the home compound.

3. Personal hygiene and cleanliness in food preparation.

4. Safe sanitation: use and maintenance of simple latrines.

Co-operation in health education activities

From the long list of subjects, *selection* of the most important local subjects is essential, and it is evident that both the community and a team of practical 'experts' in these different subjects are ideal for this selection and subsequent organization of a health education programme. For example, a schoolteacher and a school nurse can work together with the community, with the help of an agricultural extension worker, to assist in improving a home garden, in the rearing of small animals, in planning school meals, in teaching about breastfeeding, in dental health, etc.

In order to keep the educators up to date, refresher courses, workshops, and frequent meetings are needed in which an exchange of ideas and periodic evaluation of the programmes can take place.

How should health education be undertaken?

Methods

Communication. An essential aspect of health education is to be able to communicate with the audience. This usually occurs using words, signs and symbols to put over a scientific idea in a simple way. However, communication is a two-way business involving both the audience and the educator. Discussion should take place, questions should be asked on both sides, misunderstandings can be cleared up on the spot, and the subject may be brought up again in a slightly different way at a subsequent meeting to see if the message was clearly understood. The interaction between the teacher and the audience, which may consist of only one person (face-to-face education), is known as *feedback*, and this is invaluable for the educator, who will learn how to plan future talks or demonstrations. Only one message should be put over at a time, and the length of teaching should be limited to a relatively short period, possibly 15 minutes or so. Much depends on the suitability of the time chosen for the audience, on their attention span, and the surroundings in which the education is given. In some instances, classes are held in hospital clinics with a large number of people present, and the noise level is high. Under these circumstances, little will be accomplished, as there are too many distractions, and, even if the educator shouts, much of the presentation will not be heard—still less understood. The time chosen, the surroundings, as well as the topic, must be selected with care. Teaching can take place effectively under a shady tree, in a classroom, or a house. 'One-to-one' or small-group teaching is more effective, but it is more expensive, as it is time consuming and does not reach a large audience.

Which aids are used in teaching health education?

These will vary according to needs, money and local talent, such as availability of local or commercial artists, photographers etc. A number of tools have been used in the past, and newer communication methods have also developed. The term *mass media* is used to describe a number of methods which have been adopted to communicate with a small or large number of people. However, some media will be more suitable than others when dealing with illiterate audiences and with individuals who are not *pictorially literate* (e.g. not accustomed to looking at and understanding the meaning of drawings and pictures). Difficulties may occur with pictures in which people are bodily reduced in size, when they do not move, when they are shown in black and white, and when familiar clues may be missing, e.g. locally appropriate clothing, the correct village background, etc. All these must be taken into consideration when a choice of media is made. Some examples are given of various forms of techniques or media used in health education.

1. *Traditional communication forms*, e.g. *puppet shows*. These are popular, and the audience readily responds to the story which unfolds, but as they are small, seating of the audience must be carefully arranged. Live drama using *dance*

and *opera troupes* is also effective. These methods appeal to the senses of sight and hearing and are entertaining. *Role playing* is also highly effective in putting over simple messages very inexpensively. The actors can be chosen from the teaching staff or the audience, for example mothers who have become the trainers of other mothers.

2. *Visuals.* All must be tested in the actual community before use. Pictures may also be projected using an edidiascope (overhead projector) or as slides and film strips. The cost of the projector and slides etc., power and suitability, must be taken into account, and usually limit the use of these methods. Visual materials from other countries may be completely inappropriate in another area because of differences of background, clothes and general appearance.

Visuals may be subdivided into the following categories.

(a) *Books, comic books, pamphlets, flyers.* These must be suitable for the audience in terms of their literacy, and their cost must be taken into account.

(b) *Boards.* Chalk boards can be used on which messages and drawings can be imaginatively added with assistance from the audience, which promotes participation. Flannel boards and magnetic boards can also be used with flannel pictures or other pictures being added to unfold a story.

(c) *Posters and charts.* These should be simple and promote one message at a time.

(d) *Pictures.* All pictures must be studied with care before they are used, to make sure they are culturally appropriate. Individual pictures may be used, or a set of pictures may be introduced. Illiterate persons may find learning from these methods a trying task: it may be difficult to follow a sequence of pictures.

(e) *'Comic books' and fotonovellas.* These consist of stories told by photographs. These picture story books appear to be useful teaching aids for less literate or illiterate persons, and are widely used in some parts of the world.

(f) *Games.* These have become popular in more literate communities and include crossword puzzles, the 'snakes and ladders' game, the road to good breast-feeding, etc. Media which have visual appeal and entertain can be used in conjunction with real objects or live models when demonstrations are given to a large audience.

(g) *Audio media.* These include the use of radio and radio spots giving a short message (1 or 2 minutes, several times a day) as well as short lectures, tape recordings, contests etc. These appeal to the sense of hearing, also entertain, and in some countries have been very effective, especially if used at the same time as direct health education by discussion and demonstration to individuals or small groups.

(h) *Audio visuals.* These include television and sound movies. They appeal to the senses of sight and hearing, and can also entertain.

Experience has shown that a mixture of methods is best, especially small group discussion, demonstrations plus radio messages.

Miscellaneous methods

Many other activities can be carried out, such as *visits* and tours to model farms, *competitions* for the best kept compound or model garden, etc. These can be attended by local leaders, enlivened by some entertainment, and prizes given to the winners. *Health weeks* can be organized either at community or at hospital level, with stands, poster sessions, samples of nutritious foods displayed, etc. *Women's associations or clubs* are often involved in these activities, which must be planned some time ahead with permission from local representatives in the community, either in villages or in cities.

International assistance

As well as government departments, assistance may also be available from some international organisations such as UNICEF, USAID, and many non-governmental agencies, e.g. Save the Children Fund, CARE, etc., which may assist in providing materials, preparation of fotonovellas, radio spots, etc.

Health education, to be effective, must be carefully thought out, adapted to the needs of the country, culturally appropriate, and consistent between different groups. It must make families feel the need for change. It must also involve co-operation with concerned people in the community.

21
Immunization

J. Paget Stanfield

A person who is *immune* to a disease is one who is protected against that disease by means of *antibodies* circulating in his blood or present in the cells of the tissues of his body.

Immunity may be *passive* or *active*.

1. *Passive immunity*. The antibodies may be given to the child ready made, as in serum given to patients who are ill with diphtheria or tetanus. In congenital immunity, the baby receives antibodies from the mother through the placenta. The antibodies pass into the baby's blood and help to protect against infections such as measles and malaria. They slowly disappear from the baby's body, but may be present even up to the age of 1 year. Antenatal immunization of mothers against tetanus protects the newborn baby against neonatal tetanus. Another very important source of antibodies is breast milk; colostrum in particular contains large amounts of antibodies. Most of the antibodies in colostrum and breast milk remain within the baby's intestine, coating the surface of the lining cells and not being absorbed. Thus they prevent bacteria and viruses from sticking to the lining of the intestines and finding their way into the cells and bloodstream. This is the reason why breast-fed babies suffer much less from diarrhoea and other infectious diseases.

2. *Active immunity*. In this, the child makes his own antibodies. In order to start the production of antibodies, it is necessary for the person to be infected with the disease or given a vaccine which contains the bacteria or their products in a harmless form. Active immmunization, whether brought about by illness or vaccines, lasts a long time, sometimes throughout life.

201

Active immunization

Two types of vaccine are made, 'live' and 'dead'. The live vaccines contain the bacteria or virus (antigens) made harmless yet still able to infect the body and stimulate it to produce antibodies. These will then protect against the harmful form of the germ. Live vaccines produce a very mild infection of the body: a single pustule in the case of smallpox and BCG vaccines; a slight 24-hour fever with measles vaccine; a completely unnoticeable intestinal infection in the case of oral poliomyelitis vaccine. Providing the live vaccine produces infection or 'takes', one dose is sufficient to produce immunity. With live poliomyelitis vaccine, three doses are usually given because the vaccine contains three different types of poliomyelitis virus and one or two of these may infect the intestine at each dose.

The 'dead' vaccines are made either from killed bacteria or viruses or from their toxic products which have been made harmless and are called 'toxoids'. They usually have to be given at least twice before the body can build up a satisfactory immunity, and always have to be given by some form of injection. Immunity from both these types of vaccines is never complete, though it is much stronger with some than with others. For instance, whooping cough vaccine may not give a very strong protection but may still help to make any subsequent infection much milder than it would have been without the vaccine. The immunity from vaccines needs to be built up at intervals for a few years by further 'booster' doses, usually single.

Failure of a vaccine to protect an individual child may be due to a number of reasons. The vaccine may no longer be 'antigenic' so that it does not stimulate the body to produce antibodies. With a live vaccine, this may happen if the vaccine fails to 'take', which can occur if the vaccine is no longer alive. Most live vaccines are killed very easily by changes of temperature, such as might occur if they are left out of the refrigerator for a long time. This is particularly true of measles vaccine. Vaccines must be kept constantly cold throughout the chain of storage and transport which they have to pass through before reaching the child. Breaks in this 'cold chain', as it has come to be called, may be due to a batch of vaccine being left out of a refrigerator after delivery to a Ministry of Health depot or to a hospital or health centre. It could happen as a result of the breakdown of the refrigerating system. Great care must be taken to try to avoid this happening, and it is always better to have a refrigerator which can run on two different sources of power. There are some recent WHO publications which give very practical advice about this.*

Live vaccines are also damaged by sunlight, which is especially likely to happen after they have been prepared (reconstituted) for injection in the clinic or at the school. Vaccines should always be kept in the shade. They can also be affected by detergents or antiseptics in syringes which have not been properly cleaned or rinsed.

Even in the best circumstances, vaccines eventually lose their power and it is very important to look at the date of expiry on the container. This is the date after which the manufacturers cannot guarantee the power of the vaccine. Vaccines which are found to be expired should, if possible, be returned, still refrigerated, to the central store for testing. If there is no alternative, they may be used if they are within a few months after the expiry date. There is no danger that they may be harmful under these circumstances. The chances that they will fail to protect increase the longer the interval after the expiry date.

Live vaccines for injection should be used on the same day that they are reconstituted for injection, that is, after the water (diluent) has been added. Oral poliomyelitis vaccine can be used after opening until the vial is all used up, so long as it is returned to the refrigerator after clinic and kept in the shade.

* Information can be obtained from E.P.I. (Expanded Programme of Immunization) Section, World Health Organization, 1211 Geneva 27, Switzerland.

Vaccines may lose their power within the body before antibodies have been produced. This may be because antibodies from the mother are still strong enough to neutralize the vaccine. Measles vaccine, as an example, cannot be given until after at least 9 months of age to ensure that the vast majority of babies are effectively actively immunized.

Sometimes other infections make the vaccine ineffective. If a child with diarrhoea is given oral poliomyelitis vaccine, the bacteria or viruses causing the diarrhoea do not allow the poliomyelitis vaccine to stick to the gut wall and infect the body. So the vaccine fails 'to take'.

In severe malnutrition, protection produced by vaccine may also be more severe. For these reasons, ideally it is better to give passive immunity if severely malnourished children need protection. This is usually not possible owing to the cost of preparing the necessary amount of antibody, and in practice it is better to wait a few days until the child is better nourished before actively immunizing him.

Mothers may complain that in spite of vaccination, their children developed the illness. There are other infections which may closely resemble measles and whooping cough, for instance. They are usually much milder illnesses and do not last nearly as long, but it is sometimes difficult, even for an expert, to distinguish such milder attacks. One way which has been used to prevent loss of confidence amongst the public over a measles vaccine programme is to tell mothers that the vaccine will protect against severe measles.

Vaccines are now routinely available for mass campaigns against the following diseases.

Tuberculosis (BCG)	Into the skin (intradermal or multipuncture injection)
Diphtheria	Injection— either
Tetanus	subcutaneous or
Whooping cough	intradermal; usually these are available in one vaccine
Measles	Injection

Poliomyelitis	Injection or oral
Typhoid (TAB)	Injection
Yellow fever	Injection

Protection is now available against many more infections with vaccines which are becoming less costly and have fewer side-effects every year.

Recent effective vaccines include rabies, many types of influenza, mumps, rubella (German measles), chickenpox, pneumococcus, and meningococcus. Vaccines have been produced and are still being tested against hepatitis, malaria, and cholera (for which there is still no very effective protection by immunization). There are still many infections for which no satisfactory vaccine has yet been produced. The most needed of these vaccines are those which could protect against diarrhoeal infections and malaria.

Tuberculosis (p.135). The BCG vaccine contains a harmless variety of tubercle bacilli, and is given by intradermal injection by syringe or jet injector. About three weeks after injection, a small painless pustule appears which bursts and discharges slightly for about 3 weeks and then heals up, leaving a very small, depressed scar. In some countries, BCG is offered to all children and is usually given at birth or during the primary immunization course, starting at the age of 2 months and again at school age. Previous tuberculin testing is not necessary at least up to the end of primary school age. Vaccination with BCG should always be given to child contacts of tuberculous adults if they are tuberculin negative. If the child has already had a recent primary tuberculous infection, the reaction to BCG vaccination will occur within a few days, producing a large pustule and leaving a larger scar.

Diphtheria. This may not appear as a common infection in most tropical rural areas, but may be common and severe among people living in towns. Infection of skin ulcers occurs quite regularly and is often overlooked. This may be one reason why it is not recognized as much as it should be.

Immunization against diphtheria can very easily be given together with that for whooping cough and tetanus.

Whooping cough (p.165). This is an important cause of death and ill health among children. Congenital immunity against whooping cough is very slight so that whooping cough is *particularly dangerous to young babies* and they should be immunized as early as possible. Some years ago, the vaccine was suspected as being the possible cause of brain damage in a number of children. On very careful investigation, this suspicion was not confirmed and present vaccines are safe and effective.

Tetanus (p.161). This is a common and severe infection in many parts of the world, especially in the neonatal period. It does not appear in epidemics as the infection is not passed on from person to person, but arises from contamination of wounds, ulcers, infection of the ear and umbilical stump. It is very easy to protect people against tetanus at the same time as against whooping cough and diphtheria.

Triple vaccine. This contains killed whooping-cough bacteria and the toxoids of tetanus and diphtheria. Three initial intramuscular injections of 0.5 ml* of triple vaccine are necessary to provide immunization against diphtheria, whooping cough and tetanus. For children under 3 months of age, the dose should be halved. The first two doses should be given as soon as possible after the baby is 2 months old, at least a month and preferably not longer than 3 months apart. A third dose can be given after a similar interval but is best delayed for 6 months after the second dose, when it can be given with measles vaccine after the baby is 9 months old. A fourth 'booster' injection should be given later on when the child starts school. It is only necessary then for diphtheria and tetanus toxoid to be given. However, in most places this double vaccine is not available and triple should be given.

The vaccine produces a local hot, tender swelling,

* Always look at the ampoule of vaccine first to be sure of the standard dose. This varies with different manufacturers.

especially during the following night. It disappears within 2 or 3 days. With the swelling, mild fever and loss of appetite are often present for the first 12 to 24 hours. Very occasionally, especially in infants prone to febrile convulsions, this fever may be sufficient to set off such a convulsion. The vaccine should not be given if the infant or child has a fever. If there is a history of convulsions, care has to be taken with triple vaccine, but it is probably better to give rather than withhold it and risk the much more serious possibility of such convulsions in the event of whooping cough itself. If the vaccine is given to such a child, it is important to instruct the mother to keep the temperature as near normal as possible during the 24 hours following the dose, using either aspirin or paracetamol (see dosage tables).

Poliomyelitis. Immunization against poliomyelitis may be given by subcutaneous injection of killed virus or by giving the harmless vaccine by mouth, usually by drops or with sugar. It is very important that the person receives the correct number of doses recommended for the type of vaccine used. The vaccine given by mouth is probably the most suitable for children in the tropics as it is easy to give and cheap.

It is not quite so easy to produce a good antibody response to poliomyelitis when given by mouth, especially in heavily populated tropical areas. This may be due to other infections which prevent the vaccine 'taking', and for this reason the oral vaccine should not be given to anyone who has acute diarrhoea. Antibodies to poliomyelitis are excreted in breast-milk, especially in colostrum. They protect the infant against poliomyelitis, but also may prevent the vaccine from taking. This is only a problem in the first 2 or 3 weeks of life. It is probably best to try to wait an hour or more following a dose of oral polio before giving a breast-feed. More than three doses of oral polio vaccine have been given to try to make sure all three vaccines take. It is certainly not worth giving more than five doses at monthly intervals. The killed vaccine may become preferred in the future, especially if a combined vaccine (quadruple vaccine) with diptheria, tetanus and whooping cough becomes cheap. Poliomyelitis vaccine should be given at the same time as each of the doses of triple vaccine from the age of 2 months.

Typhoid (TAB). Typhoid immunization is not often given to very young children because it sometimes causes severe reactions. It is more often used in epidemics, but offers only partial protection. The vaccine can be given by intradermal injection (jet injector), when it produces a much less severe reaction.

Measles. Measles is so infectious that eradication would demand that at least three-quarters of the non-immune population was made immune. The remaining non-immune people would then be protected by an umbrella immunity called 'herd' immunity. Herd immunity can only be maintained if at least three-quarters of all babies reaching 1 year of age are immunized. Failing this, herd immunity will cease and epidemics of measles will continue. Few countries have yet been able to achieve this level of immunity, and eradication of measles is a long way off.

There are four useful and less expensive ways of using measles vaccine.

1. Controlling infection in a local community. The vaccine can be used to control measles in a local community such as a town or city or island where the infection is frequent and severe and malnutrition is common.

2. Preventing institutional infection. Measles infection can be stopped in an institution such as a hospital ward, nutritional rehabilitation unit, orphanage or residential school by vaccinating every new admission. This immediately protects the new child from catching the infection from the children already in the institution.

3. Protecting at-risk children. Children in poor health can be protected against severe measles and its bad effects — in particular underweight malnourished children, children with sickle-cell anaemia, and children recovering from tuberculosis.

4. Gaining the confidence of community leaders. The

vaccine can be used for those children whose mothers want them protected against measles. These mothers are often the leaders of their community; their confidence in measles vaccination is very important in teaching other mothers when the vaccine is cheap enough to give routinely in all clinics.

Measles vaccine should not be given before 9 months of age as at this time the child is still protected by antibodies passively obtained from his mother. There is no need to give the vaccine to children after 3 years of age as most are by then protected.

Yellow fever. This disease is not usually important from the point of view of child health. Immunization with harmless yellow fever virus is given by means of a single intramuscular injection, which should be repeated every 6 years for the international certificate which is needed for people travelling abroad. It should not be given to babies under the age of 12 months as it can, though rarely does, produce brain inflammation (encephalitis).

Smallpox. Since the last edition of this book, smallpox has been eradicated from the world. The virus survives only in one or two reference laboratories throughout the world. So the first vaccine to be used has become the first vaccine not to be needed anymore. The hope is that more and more vaccines will be unnecessary for the same reason. This has happened in some countries where infections such as tuberculosis have become almost unknown. Vaccination with BCG is now no longer routinely given in many European countries.

Jet injectors (Fig. 21.1). These instruments are being more and more widely used nowadays as they become cheaper and more reliable, though they are still not in routine use in most clinics. There are two types. The intramuscular injector, operated by means of an extremely powerful foot pump, shoots a jet of the solution through the skin into the subcutaneous tissue. These injectors are too expensive for the ordinary clinics and are used mostly in mass campaigns. The intradermal jet injector is about the size of a pen torch, and is

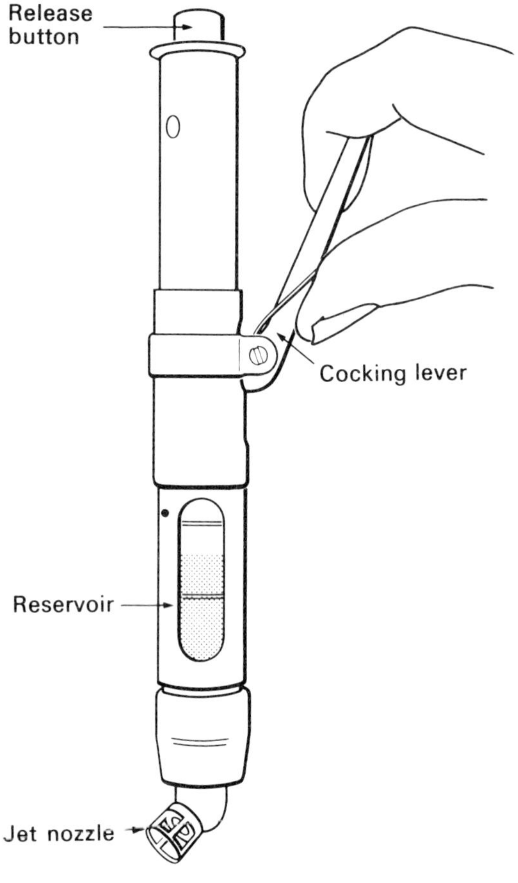

Fig. 21.1 The jet injector. *These small jet injectors are now being widely used. This model will inject 0.1 ml.

* Information on this and other types of jet injector is available from Schuco International London Ltd., Halliwick Court Place, Woodhouse Road, London N12, England.

relatively cheap. It introduces the vaccine into the skin by means of a fine jet. No needles are required and the injector is easy and quick to use. Smallpox, BCG, triple vaccine (DPT), TAB, and yellow fever vaccines can all be given by this method.

Suggested schedule (see p.213).

Immunization in the maternal and child health services

Antenatal clinics and maternity wards

In areas where tetanus neonatorum is common, the disease can be prevented by immunizing mothers against tetanus during pregnancy. Two or three doses of tetanus toxoid are given at monthly or greater intervals from the third or fourth month of pregnancy. If the mother has been immunized before, only one dose is necessary. This procedure does not, of course, replace the continuous education on umbilical hygiene which will eventually, when successful, make immunization unnecessary.

Neonatal immunization

The newborn infant is protected against many of the common childhood infections by reason of the passive transfer of antibodies from the mother by way of the placenta, colostrum and breast-milk. The duration of this protection varies from one infection to another. Active immunization is therefore not given at birth, but is delayed for a time, depending on the disappearance of passive immunity. An exception to this is BCG. There are some infections, such as tuberculosis, against which little or no immunity seems to be passed on to the infant, even though the mother may have some immunity herself.

Young-child clinics

In countries such as the UK, where most children are taken to welfare clinics, the national immunization campaign is usually based on these clinics. Diphtheria has become very uncommon in these countries since immunization became a routine procedure at child welfare clinics.

As with all the services provided at the young-child clinic, it is essential to keep records of every immunization given. In the case where the mother is given the record card, this will ensure that if she visits another clinic, her child will not be over-immunized. The only records necessary at the clinic itself will be the number immunized and whether these were first, second or third visits. If records are kept at the clinic, the mother ought also to be given a simple card in which the immunizations given to her child are noted and dated.

In a tropical country, in towns, or where there are health centres covering defined areas, a national or regional immunization campaign can also be based on the young-child clinics (p.224). In tropical rural areas where only a small proportion of the children can attend these clinics, the development of mobile clinics has answered this problem in one or two areas. All the equipment and educational material is packed in a vehicle staffed by medical auxiliaries and a health nurse. The vaccines are taken in a cold box or Thermos. By reaching out from the base medical units, as near as 3 miles, if possible, from every rural home, and by careful co-operation with the local community leaders who must be made to feel part of the campaign, a very satisfactory number of children can be protected. These mobile clinics can not only immunize, but also do other work of a young-child clinic. Immunization certainly helps to induce parents to bring their children to young-child clinics.

Suggested schedule of immunization for developing countries

Time	Vaccine	Route	Remarks
Antenatal first visit	Tetanus toxoid (alum adsorbed)	i.m.	1 ml doses at least 1 month apart
7th-8th month of pregnancy	Tetanus toxoid (alum adsorbed)	i.m.	
Birth	BCG	Intradermal	Only feasible in a large maternity unit due to wastage of multidose ampoules
6–8 weeks	DPT (triple vaccine alum adsorbed)	i.m.	Half standard dose under 3 months. Intradermal DPT has been given with entirely satisfactory results as far as the diphtheria and tetanus components are concerned in a dose of 0.1–0.2 ml
	Poliomyelitis (trivalent)	Oral	
	BCG	Intradermal	Standard sites for the country should be maintained. The vaccine can be given by jet injector intradermally

Time	Vaccine	Route	Remarks
10–12 weeks	DPT (triple vaccine alum adsorbed)	i.m.	BCG vaccination is read. If no visible reaction, repeat
	Poliomyelitis (trivalent)	Oral	
14–16 weeks	A third monthly dose of DPT and oral poliomyelitis vaccines can be given but may be unnecessary.		
9 months to 1 year	DPT (triple vaccine alum adsorbed)	i.m.	
	Poliomyelitis (trivalent)	Oral	
	Measles	i.m.	Most workers still recommend the full dose of 1000 TCD_{50} intramuscularly, usually in 0.5 ml when reconstituted. Intradermal vaccination is still too uncertain to be advised on a large scale. Frequent monitoring of the vaccine dose entering the skin is necessary.
5-6 years	Tetanus toxoid (alum adsorbed)	i.m.	
School age			
	Poliomyelitis (trivalent)	Oral	
	BCG	Intradermal	

22

Maternal and child health services

F. John Bennett

Child health services are always part of a system of care that covers the whole cycle of child-bearing and child-rearing in the family. It is better, therefore, to use a term such as maternal and child health (MCH) services. In some parts of the world, they may be called family health services.

Primary health care is the essential health care made easily accessible to all individuals, children and families in the community. This is done with participation from the community and it is linked to other aspects of development such as education and agriculture. This health care at community level is supported for referral, supervision and supplies by more complex health services provided in units such as health centres and hospitals. Primary health care is carried out by community health workers who live in the community and are properly trained to carry out the essential services which the community needs and can afford. Primary health care includes at least:

> maternal and child care including family planning
> promotion of proper nutrition and food supply
> adequate safe water and basic sanitation
> immunization
> prevention and control of locally endemic diseases
> health education
> treatment of common diseases and injuries and provision of basic drugs.

This primary health care based in the community can be quite simple, but it is the first part of a system which allows for referral to more trained and more specialized staff in bigger units. For example, the primary health care worker might be a traditional birth attendant who has received training at a nearby health centre and who is able to care for a mother with a normal pregnancy and delivery, and who can then advise on the care of the newborn or young infant. The primary health worker is able to refer mothers and infants to the nearest health centre for more sophisticated services.

The integrated family health service

Most health centres, clinics, hospital out-patient services or mobile clinics now provide all the components of maternal and child health and family planning (or spacing) services at the same time and place daily. This is possible if each member of the staff has been trained in all these aspects, or if the staff has been trained as a team. The elements involved in MCH services can be described separately, but it is always preferable that they be provided together—on the 'super-market' basis where the mother comes with her family and obtains what she needs. This might be antenatal care for herself, weighing and advice for the 2-year-old child, and treatment for the 4-year-old child with a fever.

The different elements of MCH care

Antenatal care

The aim of antenatal care is to have a healthy mother produce a healthy baby. Education of the mother and father alone or in groups about nutrition, childbirth and child-rearing, ar-rangements for the treatment of illness in the mother and for a safe delivery, are all parts of antenatal work which can have a helpful and long-term effect on the baby. Antenatal services are usually held at clinics or hospitals so as to be continuous with the midwifery service and young-child service.

Mobile MCH clinics often combine looking after the preg-nant mother at the same time as caring for her young children. Combined services thus save the mother having to make many journeys. One of the main purposes of antenatal services is to select 'high-risk' mothers who must have skilled delivery in an institution. High-risk cases would include young or old mothers, first babies, mothers who have had many babies, twins, mothers with previous difficult labours, very short women and women with complications or medical conditions such as anaemia. Immunization against tetanus can be given to mothers in antenatal clinics to prevent tetanus neonatorum.

Antenatal care should also provide the pregnant women with extra iron and folate, if necessary, to prevent anaemia, and with chloroquine to prevent malaria in endemic areas.

Midwifery service

This is concerned with the health of the baby and mother at the period of the birth. In rural areas, hospital delivery is usually reserved for abnormal labour or first births, whereas normal childbirth takes place at home, perhaps conducted by an unskilled village midwife (such as the *dai* of India), but preferably by a trained midwife (domiciliary service). The quality of care before and at birth can influence the number of babies suffering from infections (including tetanus) and birth injuries (especially brain damage) which can have serious permanent effects on the child.

Postnatal care

In an MCH clinic providing postnatal care, both mother and baby are examined and treated, if necessary, for any abnormal condition discovered. This is usually about 4–6 weeks after the birth of a baby. The mother is given advice and the baby is perhaps started with immunization, and an arrangement is made for future attendance at a young-child clinic.

Family planning clinics

In some countries, family spacing is the term which is preferred as it is more in keeping with traditional practices. In order to space their pregnancies at the best intervals and, when desired, to limit the number of children to what the family can afford, parents need advice. The first advice may come from the primary health worker, who then refers the mother to the MCH centre where she can get expert advice and help. Sometimes these services are provided by voluntary or private agencies, but it is always better if they are undertaken as part of the normal care provided for families at MCH centres, antenatal clinics, postnatal clinics or maternity units.

Premature unit

Premature or pre-term babies (p.42) need special care, and many hospitals with a large midwifery department also have a 'premature unit' with staff trained in this work.

Newborn

Because there are special risks (infection, bleeding, maternal ill health and feeding difficulties) in the newborn period (p.27), most midwifery departments prefer to look after the mother and baby for a few days, although at present this is not possible in many tropical regions because of a shortage of maternity beds. It is desirable to visit the mother in her home in the first month of the baby's life, but with few staff this may have to be limited to 'high-risk neonatals', e.g. small babies, mothers with some illness, twins.

The maternal and child health services which guard the baby during pregnancy and in the newborn period may be organized by the government of the country or by the community. They are usually made up either of hospitals (together with their out-patient departments), or of health centres with a staff of home-visiting midwives and health visitors (or similar personnel). This type of service may also arise as a result of the efforts of such voluntary organizations as the Red Cross or Women's Clubs. Care of the newborn in many countries is now helped by having primary health workers living in and supported by the community.

Young child care

This aims at preventing illness, promoting health and providing treatment of minor ailments of the child during the
first 5 years of life. Important aspects are immunization,
nutritional surveillance, and guidance and education of the
mother. Any disabilities or handicaps should also be identified so as to assist the mother and to start rehabilitation.

Mobile MCH clinics

In some countries with great distances, a scattered population
and few trained staff, mobile clinics might be organized.
These visit villages or clinic sites once a month and provide
MCH services to families. They are especially useful for
bringing immunization to areas without refrigeration for stor-
ing vaccines. Because of the increasing cost of transport,
mobile clinics are, however, now less important than static
clinics and primary health workers. However, the supervisory
management team for a district with a primary health care
programme may still need to be mobile.

Hospital wards and out-patient departments

These are required to treat seriously ill children and to return
children to full activity (rehabilitate) after illness.

In most tropical peasant communities where breast-feeding
is the rule, it is essential that the mother be admitted to
hospital with her child and provision should be made for this.
This also supplies a valuable opportunity for health education
for mothers (p.190), prevents the child from being frightened
by being separated, and permits mothers to help with the care
of their children.

Both young-child clinics and hospitals may be run by the
same organization (e.g. the central government, the local
government or mission) and, in this case, there should be a
very close link between them as regards the work done,
methods used and the staff employed. An example of this
would be when the young-child clinic staff would organize a

programme of health education for mothers in a hospital ward.

Nutrition rehabilitation

This service is sometimes organized in centres or units for the care and treatment of moderately undernourished children. The buildings may be simply constructed of local material and situated near to the village. The unit is run by a nurse or an auxiliary, together with help from the mothers. Children are fed on low-cost local food mixtures (multimixes) prepared by the mothers who can observe their own children's improvement and weight gains. Instead of being carried out in a residential unit, nutritional rehabilitation can also be done within the community through a women's organization on a co-operative basis.

Research units

This type of unit, often specializing in certain children's diseases (e.g. malnutrition or tuberculosis) has a big part to play in solving the particular difficulties found in different countries. Their successful methods must, however, be made known to rural hospitals and health centres.

Health services for nursery schools

In the few, but increasing, places where these exist, advantage can be taken of the gathering of a group of preschool children—an age which is otherwise little seen by medical staff, as a 4-year-old is too big to carry and too small to walk long distances to a health clinic. Immunization, periodic examinations, and nutritional improvement by food supplements are three important aspects of health assistance for this age group.

School health services (p.238)

Handicapped children

There are children who, because of some disadvantage, such as lameness, blindness or deafness, are not able to do what normal children can do. They are a problem in poor communities as they may require long and expensive treatment before being able to become useful citizens.

Loss of special sense, such as hearing or sight, is sometimes dealt with in a school for the deaf or blind where the child can be taught to overcome his handicap and eventually earn his own living. Mentally backward children may also benefit from special schools which let them proceed at their own slower rate of development. A service for finding, treating and teaching handicapped children (due to poliomyelitis, tuberculosis, congenital defects and accidents) will save a lot of them from becoming a burden to their families and to the country.

Orphans and other children without the care and love of their parents are more of a problem in some societies than in others, and places for their care may be necessary. In such orphanages, however, it is always important that there be homely, close personal contact between the children and some adults on the staff. Foster parents may be useful in providing temporary or permanent homes for orphans, especially in towns where this problem is increasing. Legal adoption of babies is sometimes done through an organization, e.g. a church or voluntary society.

Services for handicapped children and children deprived of family life are often started late in a country's development, and the first stages might be begun by voluntary effort. It is best for this service to be developed together with those responsible for the schools and the medical services of a country.

Any services developed must be simple and inexpensive and should aim at training people to fit into the local community.

Child guidance clinics

Emotional   disturbances   and   failures   to   fit   into   the community's way of life (behaviour problems) occur throughout childhood and include bedwetting, thumb-sucking, refusal to go to school, and juvenile delinquency. The commonness of this type of problem is not known in most tropical countries.

A health service may deal with such problems by organizing child guidance clinics where parents and children can be advised. Social workers and health visitors can also do valuable work in this type of problem because of their knowledge of the family background and its effects on behaviour problems.

Youth clubs

These provide harmless and useful outlets for the energy of older children. Such clubs are also valuable for health education purposes and for such activities as games which improve the health of children.

CHILD to child health services

There is an increasing awareness that older children can help to improve the health of other children by greater involvement in simple health activities. These activities within a village or within families can be stimulated by active learning in the schools or through women's organizations.

Community development, agricultural extension services, and community schools

Primary health care is most successful when there is co-ordinated action for development by several ministries. It is not possible to think of health for all children without improvements in food production, in water supply, in education, in housing etc., as all these are also related to health. Therefore, the extension workers from other ministries and the teachers from the schools should work together with health workers in a community to promote health and prevent disease, especially in mothers and children.

Organization of child health services

In most countries, all the health services mentioned have been built up separately and slowly and through many groups—government, religious organizations, the community, industry and voluntary organizations. It is important, however, to see them all as part of the child health services and as part of the same attempt to improve all aspects of child health.

Many countries have a senior specialist in child health, or maternal and child health, in the Ministry of Health who co-ordinates all these services and ensures that they receive the correct emphasis.

International organizations

In most parts of the world, such international organizations as UNICEF, WHO and FAO are playing a part in assisting governments to develop their child health services.

Governments are assisted by FAO to improve nutrition by better farming and fisheries, and by WHO to improve child health by supplying experts, by assisting in training programmes, etc.

The United Nations Children's Fund (UNICEF) co-operates with government programmes in health (especially primary health care, with an emphasis on maternal and child health), education, agriculture, water development, village technology, women's activities, preschool centres, and in urban improvement projects. It supplies drugs, vaccines, equipment for maternal and child health services, transport, and helps in training programmes. Both UNICEF and the International Red Cross also help in emergencies and with problems of refugee children due to wars and political disturbances.

23
Young-child clinics

J. Paget Stanfield

Young-child clinics are one of the ways in which health services are delivered to infants and children. They are centres within and around which primary care is organized and delivered and where mothers make their first contact with the health and medical services. They are often combined with maternal and family health care services and linked with community development, agricultural, marketing and educational centres for the local community. Young-child clinics aim to keep infants and young children well and to allow them to reach their fullest potential. They do this in a number of different ways which include the following.

1. Entering into the life of the people, encouraging and guiding desires and activities which improve their health and quality of life.

2. Recording births and deaths and observing and recording the state of health and development of mothers and children within the community. This is the beginning of recording vital statistics (see below).

3. Identifying the priority problems of ill health amongst children, their causes and effects and possible remedies within the community: this is called community diagnosis.

4. Detecting families who are at special risk of developing ill-health (mental or physical) and situations which may predispose to breakdown of health, and making particular efforts to prevent this happening.

5. Detecting early signs of disease in the individual child or within the community, and trying to prevent and reverse the process.

6. Curing illness as early and as completely as possible, either at the clinic or by referral to hospital.

7. Rehabilitating sick, injured, deprived or handicapped

infants and children as rapidly and completely as possible.

8. Co-operating as far as possible with any other agencies, healing or caring, that are committed to building up the quality of life in the community.

At the young-child clinic primary care level, there are no divisions between cure and prevention, between treatment and rehabilitation, between the individual, the family and the community. They all form part of the work of the staff of the clinic. How can such a wide variety of tasks be managed effectively? There are three main requirements.

1. *Training*. The staff need to be well trained in a number of different disciplines so that they know what they can do themselves, and to whom to refer for advice or help.

2. *Teamwork*. The staff must try to work as a team. A team needs a leader, and each member has a specific part to play in the whole unit. The team will need to meet fairly frequently to discuss problems, successes and failures and what to do about them.

3. *Work satisfaction*. Finally, people are more important than posts. However well organized, a clinic will only run well if there is satisfaction and purpose in the work of each member of staff. Support and encouragement will be needed from the central administration, not only with supplies, but also with visits and organized refresher programmes at regular intervals.

In practice the every-day work of the staff of the young-child clinic will include the following.

Education

Of the parents in groups or individually (pp.190, 234).

In all education at children's clinics, it is important to be practising what is being preached, especially in the matter of cleanliness, toilet facilities and nutrition. Some clinics have become actively involved and identified in their work with the local community. A small vegetable garden, hens, rabbits or even a cow will supply the right sort of food which can be cooked at the clinic times in an improved kitchen. If the cost of this activity is always kept within the income level of the community, it will enable the teaching to be much more realistic. A parents' club can be formed, and self-help schemes encouraged.

In schools

Probably the most important people to influence are the school children as they are the future generation, and many will be parents in a few short years. Links with the teaching staff of the local primary and secondary schools could lead to visits by clinic staff to the school for teaching or demonstration. Some schools are very active in nutrition, food preparation and small-holding agriculture. There may be a school farm. The children can be invited to the clinic to see for themselves babies being weighed, one or two ill babies being treated, weight charts, care of the newborn etc.

Supervision and treatment of children

1. Observing and recording child's progress.
2. Weight and measurements.
3. Clinical examination.
4. Treatment.
5. Availability of free or cheap foods.
6. Immunization.

The way the clinic is run will depend on the kind of staff and equipment available and the attitude of the local people. In some places there will be very few trained staff and very little equipment, perhaps not even scales for weighing. In some places, clinics will be so overcrowded that it will be impossible to give individual attention. Sometimes the clinic may be mainly for treatment of sick children; sometimes it may be more like a health education meeting, with very little available in the way of supervision and treatment of the children.

Observing and recording a child's progress

When the children are attending the clinic regularly, their progress can be observed and any abnormality or disease diagnosed and treated at the earliest possible stage or, if possible, prevented from occurring. In order to find out whether the child is progressing as he should, it is necessary to keep careful records of the child's weight and other physical signs observed at each attendance.

Record cards are as various in their form as clinics. The best one in the experience of many is a stiff, folded card, on one side of which there is a chart of normal weight. If the child's weight is recorded on this graph, a poor gain or fall in weight can be seen at a glance. On the other side, there is a space for recording notes, immunization etc. (p.212). These cards are best given to the mother, if possible in a plastic folder. Records kept at the clinic should be mainly numbers and types of illness seen, of immunizations, of health education topics, of child-spacing methods, etc. It is usually necessary to keep copies of records of patients who are 'at risk' or actually sick. A list of indications of 'at risk' children needs to be made. This list could include children whose weight is found to lie below the lowest line of the weight chart; whose weight falls below the child's usual weight path; who show one or more signs of malnutrition, or who are paler than usual. Copies of the records of these children are then kept at the clinic and the children may then be followed up separately at an 'at-risk' clinic until their weight catches up to its normal path, or until the 'risk' indication is no longer present. These records, if kept, can indicate the success of nutrition rehabilitation from the weight 'catch-ups' and, if the child fails to attend, the address can be used for a home visit.

The numerical records of the clinic can be charted on a graph week by week. This can be very helpful in showing when an epidemic is beginning (for instance of measles or diarrhoeal disease), so that something perhaps can be done soon enough to prevent it spreading (such as measles or

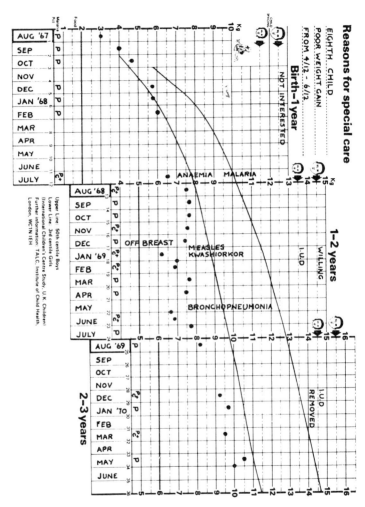

Fig. 23.1 The *Road to Health* chart. *This is now suggested as a standard pattern. The objective will be to see that the child increases in weight regularly and, as shown on this chart, there is usually evidence many months before a child develops malnutrition. The same chart can be used to identify children requiring special care, and also to encourage and supervise family planning.

228

cholera immunization). A map of the area served by the clinic also helps to show where the patients are coming from, and which homes and schools have been visited. Such a map, if kept up to date, can be very useful in teaching and explaining to visitors the work of the clinic. Good numerical records kept by every young-child clinic could be the beginning of a complete system of health statistics for the area.

Weight and measurements

Weight (Fig. 23.1)
Weighing is the simplest method of observing the child's growth. If the clinic is attached to a maternity unit, it is important to record birth weight. Low birth weight (less than 2500 g) is an indication for special care; the number of low-birth-weight babies should decrease as the health and well-being of a community rise.

In the young-child clinic, if the child's age is known, his weight can be compared with that of normal children of the same age and at the same group. If his weight is very much below that of normal children of the same age, he is probably undernourished. Even if the child's age is not known, it is possible to weigh him every time he comes to the clinic and see whether he is *gaining* weight. This is very important. If a child loses weight suddenly, he usually has some acute infection; if he fails to gain weight for several months, he is almost certainly malnourished or has some chronic infection.

The young child should be expected to gain at least the following weight: first 6 months, 340 g (¾ lb) every month; second 6 months, 450 g (1 lb) every 2 months; second year, 450 g (1 lb) every 4 months.

Method of weighing. The following must be available, otherwise it is better to run the clinic without attempting to weigh the children.

* Specimens of this card, and teaching aids that may be used with it, are available from Teaching Aids at Low Cost (TALC), Institute of Child Health, 30 Guildford Street, London WC1N 1EH.

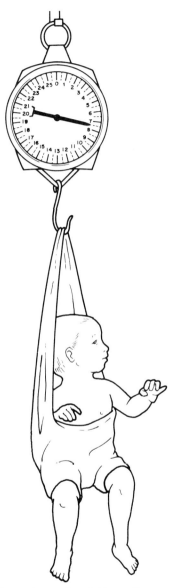

Fig. 23.2 Salter spring scale: sturdy, reliable, easily transported.

An accurate weighing machine (Figs. 23.2, 23.3 and 23.4) checked daily;
Staff who can be trained to weigh accurately;
Someone to interpret the weight record.

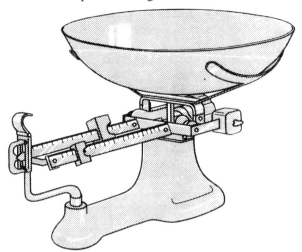

Fig. 23.3 The beam balance scale is the traditional and reliable way of weighing babies. The larger weight should record kilograms and the smaller from 0 to 1000 grams.

It is no use at all weighing children unless it is done correctly. A weighing machine is a delicate instrument and must be handled gently. If the machine is not working properly, this must be reported at once. It is useless to weigh children on a faulty machine. Always weigh the children either naked or in a single cotton garment; sweaters, towelling nappies or shoes must be removed before weighing. The weight must be charted or noted down carefully. If there is a marked or unexpected difference between it and the previous weight, it is wise to recheck the reading on the scale.

Other measurements

Height is the most accurate way of observing growth but is usually too difficult to measure accurately in a routine clinic.

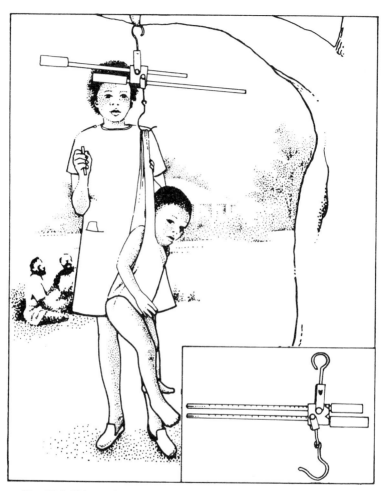

Fig. 23.4 This steelyard beam and balance instrument has been used successfully in a number of countries for weighing infants. It is suspended from a tree or a beam and is extremely portable and durable. The infant or child is hung from the bottom hook in a sack or trouser suit. The top beam is a kilogram scale and the bottom a pound scale, and the weight of the sack or trousers can be balanced before the child is weighed by one or other beam, whichever is not being used.*

* Details of weighing machines and other anthropometric equipment are available from CMS Weighing Equipment Ltd, 18 Camden High Street, London NW1 OJH.

Mid-upper-arm circumference has been used successfully at many young-child clinics to detect malnutrition; it is measured round the arm, halfway between the shoulder and the point of the elbow. It remains at about 16 cm from the age of 1 year to 5 years, and a mid-upper-arm circumference of less than 14 cm between these two ages indicates some degree of malnutrition.

Clinical examination

Ideally, this should include a full physical examination at first attendance and at intervals after this, together with such examinations as blood films, haemoglobin levels and tuberculin skin tests.

In practice, it is usually only possible to inspect the child. Inspection should include looking for the following.

1. *Signs of malnutrition.* Does he look roughly the right height and weight for his age? Are his skin, hair and muscles normal? Is he swollen or oedematous? Is he happy? If breast-fed, does he suck well and are his mother's breasts normal? Are his eyes shiny or dull and dry? Are there any foamy patches on his conjunctivae? Or do they look dry and wrinkled?

2. *Signs of abnormal or slow development.* Does he behave like a normal child of his age? Does he look interested? Are there any abnormal movements? Does he talk like other children of his age?

3. *Signs of infection.* Does his body feel hot, dry and feverish? Is his pulse rapid? Has he a cough and, if so, does he whoop? Has he any discharge from eyes, nose or ears, or ulcers in his mouth? Has he any lumps (glands) in his neck? Has he any pustules or ulcers on his scalp or skin, or any cuts or jiggers on his feet? Has he a rash or red eyes? Has he a palpable spleen?

4. *Signs of anaemia.* Do the reds of his eyes or his tongue or gums look pale, or the whites of his eyes look yellow? Is he swollen or oedematous?

5. *Signs of dehydration.* Has he diarrhoea or vomiting? Are

his eyes or fontanelle, if still open, sunken? Is his mouth dry?
Does his skin wrinkle to remain wrinkled?

Treatment

Treatment should always be available for children attending a
young-child clinic. Children who are brought to a centre
because they are acutely sick with infectious diseases (e.g.
measles) should be kept apart. A few standard tablets of
medicine (such as aspirin, chloroquine, sulphadimidine and
ferrous sulphate) can be pre-packaged in envelopes with the
dosage written on in the language of the mother. This saves
time and staff in dispensing. Children should be given the best
possible treatment as quickly as possible and told to return
home, but to come back when the child is better and then
attend clinic regularly. The main objects of treatment, apart
from curative, at the child welfare clinic are *educational* and
preventive.

At intervals, the lines of flow of the mothers and children
going through the clinic should be looked at to make sure that
waiting time for the mothers is as short as possible, and is
being used profitably in teaching and demonstration. Any
time- or labour-saving devices should be tried out and used if
successful. Sufficient and suitably low benches should be
supplied for the waiting mothers.

Educational treatment.

A child is usually brought to the clinic in the first place
because his parents think he is ill. The mother will usually ask
for medicine or an injection. Very often the child is not really
ill; what the mother needs is *advice* rather than *medicine*.
Even if the child is ill, always remember that medicine will be
of very little use unless the child is nursed and looked after
properly—and the mother must be advised how to do this. In
this way, her concern for her child will be used as a way to
teach her how to look after the child, and she will gain
experience which will be valuable to her in the future.

A good practical example of this is the child with diarrhoea who is not so dehydrated as to need admission. The mother can be seated on a low bench with room for other children with the same complaint. Next to the bench is a large container; it is better if it is similar to the type mother uses at home, like a gourd. This is filled before the clinic starts with cooled boiled water. It is covered in some way to keep off flies. A number of clean cups and teaspoons, one bottle containing sugar and another containing salt—both labelled correctly—complete the necessary 'diarrhoea rehydration kit'. The mother is shown, perhaps by the health visitor or nursing aid, how to take a cupful of boiled water and add one pinch of salt between two fingers and two teaspoonfuls of sugar. She then stirs the mixture and gives it by spoon or cup to the child. She can be left there for half an hour or so. If the child finishes the cup without vomiting, and the mother seems able to continue the drink, as most often happens, then she can be told to go home and do exactly the same at home for the next 6 hours. Then she can give diluted milk for the next 12 hours, and then go on to solids. She learns the importance of cleanliness in feeding by doing, and knows that if the child gets diarrhoea again, she should give this treatment before she brings the child to the clinic.

Preventive treatment
Minor illness (e.g. scabies) are treated to prevent serious complications (severe skin infections). Infectious conditions (e.g. diarrhoea) are treated so as to prevent them from spreading to others.

Hospital treatment
A good link should be maintained with the nearest hospital, so that the very sick children can be admitted with as little difficulty as possible.

Availability of free or cheap food
At some clinics, supplies of dried skimmed milk, or other

supplement from outside agencies, are available for distribution to children during the weaning period. Sometimes, other food supplements may be available, perhaps even grown or produced at the clinic, in which case these may be sold at low cost. When this is so, the food should, of course, be used as a means of *teaching* the parents. The parents can be shown different ways of using the milk with the child's food, and, if possible, they should be visited at home to make sure that they are using it properly. It is always important to have some food available for the treatment of malnourished children.

Immunization

Some important children's diseases such as measles, whooping cough and poliomyelitis are preventable by immunization (p.201). Sometimes immunization against these diseases will be done in young-child clinics as part of an immunization campaign in a particular area. Preventive immunizations are very important and should be given to all children attending the clinic unless there are reasons for not doing so. They should be one part of the effort towards educating the parents and helping the children.

Other activities

In many young-child clinics, an antenatal clinic and family planning advice may be available also for mothers who need or desire them. There may also be other primary care workers in community development or agriculture, either attached to the clinic or health centre or in a nearby community development or farming centre. Their advice and help in teaching can be of great value in the health centre. It can also be repaid by looking after the health of the worker's families. Leaders of the local church or mosque may be invited to become involved in the organisation of a community club which could undertake self-help health projects such as water supply, food and water for storage. Their advice could be sought to help with broken, depressed and deprived families and in adoption and fostering problems.

Line of flow at clinic

Exactly how to set about running a clinic will depend on circumstances, but the general procedure may be as follows.

While parents and children assemble, group talks and demonstrations are given. The child is weighed and the weight recorded on a card which may be kept by the mother or by the clinic. In rural clinics, the former method is the most satisfactory and realistic. The child is examined, and progress and any treatment recorded. During the examination, individual advice can be given to parents. Finally, the child is given the necessary immunizations.

If there is anyone in the clinic available for home visiting, this can be done on non-clinic days.

It is important to check stocks of food, medicines and records, so that fresh supplies can be obtained before they finish completely.

It is always welcome if there is available at the clinic, in an obvious place, a source of clean water for thirsty mothers and children.

Well-signposted toilets, of a type that could be built in an average home and kept clean and tidy, are very important not only for use but as a teaching aid.

24
School health services

F. John Bennett

Wherever there are schools for children, there is the need for some type of school health service and, at the same time, there is the possibility that something useful can be done no matter what staff and money are available.

Special need. There are six reasons for the special need for a health service for schools.

1. During this part of their lives, children are growing and developing (physically, mentally and as members of the community), so that any improvement of their health or correction of their diseases may have an effect all through their lives.

2. For many children, school is the first time they have come into contact with people outside their family. This change means journeys, exposure to infectious diseases and the competition of school life, which, in turn, carry the dangers of accidents, infections, and general physical and emotional strain.

3. The school has very good opportunities for health education which can reach not only the child, but also his home, and indeed the next generation, when the schoolchild himself grows and becomes a parent.

4. In order to benefit from school, children need good health and freedom from disease and handicaps, so that there should be some way of finding and correcting anything which might stop them being able to learn.

5. The school is always part of a community and it may be the first part in which new ideas on health will be accepted and understood and from which they can spread.

6. This school-going age group might form as much as a quarter of the whole population, so that it is clear how important a health service is for them.

238

Healthy living in schools

This is the most important way in which to begin health work in schools.

1. *Environmental hygiene.* Every school should pay attention to its water supply, disposal of excreta and of rubbish, prevention of insect breeding, and the condition of its buildings with regard to overcrowding, ventilation and lighting. Sometimes this can be done by getting the interest, and then the assistance, of the community which the school serves, for example by their supplying labour and materials for protection of the school water supply. In some countries and in most towns the school environment is controlled by laws and regulations which may say exactly the size of classrooms, the amount of window space, the number of latrines, etc. It is most important that such regulations are carried out in boarding schools or big schools because the risks of spread of infection are greater and may affect more children. Some of the people who could make a contribution to this part of school health are health inspectors, health visitors, and the teachers and school authorities themselves.

2. *School feeding.* If children are to study well throughout the day, they should have something to prevent hunger. This could be a small meal provided either by the parents or by the school, if funds are available or if they can be collected from the parents. A school meal also provides an opportunity for making sure that each child gets what might be missing from his diet, especially protein and vitamins. The foods given should always be ones that are locally suitable and can form part of the normal home diet of the child. School feeding can be used as an aid to the teaching of nutrition and new food habits and it can also be used as a lesson in agriculture, if the school has a garden which produces sufficient food for use by the pupils.

3. *The school day.* The school programme should be so planned as to contribute to the health of the child. The hours of work, the periods of play, and a feeling of happiness in the classroom all influence the growing pupil.

4. *Physical activities in the school.* Sport in schools should improve strength, endurance and agility and it should give the child opportunity to learn to work with others in a team. Sport can also help a child to learn about good health. However, it is wise to remember that physical activities should not use up too much of the calories which a child in a poor community might require for walking home. If possible, sport in schools should be related to sport in the community.

5. *Promotion of mental health in the school.* The first aim is to have happy, satisfied teachers who enjoy their work, and the second is to have pupils who are understood and who are encouraged to develop their ability to make friends and to discover what they can do best in life. In some areas the school could try to give the child some idea of the responsibilities of family living. The use of punishment in a school should be carefully considered, as it can sometimes do more damage than it does good. Too much emphasis on marks, examinations and competition can prove to be a stress for a child and can lead to symptoms such as eye, head and stomach pains—this is especially found in secondary schools and also upper primary classes.

6. *Health education.* One of the aims of education is to teach the child to improve his own health and to realize the part he can play in protecting the health of others in the community. To do this the child must be given knowledge of how the body works, of the causes and prevention of the important diseases, and of modern ideas about health services.

The school health education programme should always be fitted in with the health-education programme for the whole community, and this will usually mean working together with local staff in such departments as Agriculture and Community Development. It is also important in planning school health education to have the advice of a doctor who knows the health problems of the area.

Much of school health education can be done without special lectures, especially by having healthy surroundings at school from which the child learns by actual experience.

In short, health education must be included in the everyday

life of schoolchildren. It should not aim at changing the way of life of the local community but rather at modifying certain customs which are harmful (p.12). In health education, the emphasis must be on the child learning actively, rather than just sitting and being taught.

Some of the most important topics of health education in the school are personal cleanliness and hygiene in the home, the school, and the village; the best use of local foods; insects, worms and animals that cause disease; and the best methods of bringing up children. It is important to try to see how effective this type of health education is, and, when necessary, to change the methods used. As the foundation for some future health problems may be laid down during the school age, it is important to try to prevent these by education and guiding the children's attitudes. Smoking, promiscuous sexual behaviour, use of alcohol and drugs are activities which may start in school. Health education for schoolchildren should not be left to teachers and workers in various ministries, but should also involve parents from the community.

Prevention of disease in schoolchildren

1. *Supervision of the teacher's health.* If possible, teachers should be medically examined before employment and, if practicable, should also have periodic examinations to exclude diseases such as infectious tuberculosis.

2. *Safety and accident prevention.* The school buildings and grounds should be safe and they need frequent inspection and thought in order to prevent accidents. If an accident occurs, the reasons for it should be looked into so that similar accidents can be prevented in the future.

3. *Infectious diseases.* Immunization (p.201) against diseases such as poliomyelitis, tuberculosis, diphtheria, tetanus and typhoid can be done in the school, and quite often this can be used as a means of persuading the rest of the community to be immunized.

In most countries, children with certain infectious diseases have to be excluded from school for a period of time laid down in regulations.

4. *Prevention of common epidemic diseases.* Acute conjunctivitis, trachoma, dysentery, meningitis, scabies, ringworm and louse infestations are prevented from assuming epidemic proportions in a school by attention to environmental hygiene, by immunization, and by early diagnosis and treatment.

Diagnostic and curative services for the school

1. *Health examination and early diagnosis of abnormalities.* There is a need in every school for a continuous health observation by an alert and informed teacher, rather than occasional, medical examination of the pupils. Records should be continuous and be passed on from class to class or school to school as the child grows. If possible, parents should be present at examinations done by doctors because their observations and co-operation are needed.

The purpose of health examination of pupils is to provide doctors, parents and teachers with information concerning the growth and health of the children, to find pupils needing further examination or treatment, to correct conditions in an early stage before they affect the child, or his classmates, and, lastly, to teach the parents, children and school staff the importance of health. The teacher's place in health examination is most important because he is the one who observes the child over a long period and should be able to detect any ill-health at an early stage. The teacher in some places is also responsible for simple vision testing, weighing, examination of the skin and ears, and selection of cases for the doctor's examination.

The number of times schoolchildren can be examined medically depends on the staff available, but a useful ideal would be the examination of all children on entering or on leaving school, and also examination of any children specially referred by the teacher. However, this is seldom possible in developing countries and the main use of examinations, when done in a sample of classes, is that it is part of a 'community diagnosis', i.e. it shows what conditions are common in this age group and thus helps in the planning of suitable preventive and control measures for the whole school population.

2. *First aid.* As minor accidents are always occurring in schools, there should be a simply equipped first-aid box and someone trained in its use. Classes in first aid for children can also use this equipment.

3. *Treatment.* Arrangements for treatment of defects discovered at routine examination or for treatment of sickness occurring at school should, if possible, be made through the child's family, who should be persuaded and helped to make the best use of locally available services. For some cases, specialist treatment is necessary, and it may be possible to arrange this through the school health service, as, for example, with the treatment of handicapped children. Some large schools might have a school nurse, who is able to give simple treatments.

4. *Management of chronic conditions.* Schools can help to ensure that children on medication for conditions requiring long-term treatment, such as epilepsy and leprosy, continue to get their treatment regularly. Although there is often a stigma attached to these two diseases, teachers, supported by the health workers, can ensure that the children continue with schooling while receiving continued medical care.

Organization of school health services

In many countries, there is a medical officer either in the Ministry of Health or in the Ministry of Education who is especially concerned with school health. In other areas, this work is done by the district medical workers. The contribution of the teachers is always very important, and they can be helped if courses are held to teach them about the local health problems. Parents too must be included in local school health committees if these are started to plan improvements such as school feeding or water supplies.

25
Community involvement

P.M. Shah

In the past, health programmes in developing countries have been organized with little attention to real involvement of the community. For this reason, services offered by governmental and non-governmental agencies are often accepted without any action by people themselves, as aid or charity. Until recently, few attempts have been made to encourage community involvement. The greater the participation of the community in the development of primary health care (p.215), the greater will be their eagerness (motivation) to accept and use these services, the smaller will be the need for expensive curative care in hospitals, and the smaller will be the risk of unnecessary ill-health and death, especially among children. Health workers should have a good understanding of community development programmes and be able to help and to encourage an attitude of 'self-help' and real action by the population, which is very often willing and able to contribute, even though poor and illiterate.

Scope

Community involvement can apply to many health activities, extending from discussing together, making decisions on priorities, carrying out programmes and supervising them, and measuring how useful they have been. This involvement may be limited to the local elite or leaders, but, ideally, it should include all men, women and young people interested in improving their community. The influence that the community can have on making decisions can extend from the village through the provincial authorities to the national government, as well as to the political party or parties of the country.

Community development programmes should encourage ideas and plans by villagers rather than impose upon communities plans from outside agencies. Local initiative has to be based on the identification of 'felt needs' and of the steps to be taken to improve matters, partly by 'self-help' in which the community helps in various ways, including manpower, labour and finance (within its usually very limited capacity), while the government and outside agencies provide part of the money needed, technical guidance, supplies not available locally, training, supervision and referral services, and help to fit these activities into larger regional and national programmes.

Experiences with community involvement

The value of the community involvement in programmes is highest with mothers and young children. Many activities have been carried out by the community in some developing countries and many more are being encouraged.

Manpower

A most important part of community involvement is by the use of individuals from the same village as primary health care workers. Experiences from many countries have shown that simply trained, local health workers, even when illiterate, can successfully organize and carry out basic maternal and child health programmes as part of primary health care. Important mortality rates (such as infant mortality, p.1 and 1–4-year mortality, p.2), the frequency (incidence) of malnutrition and of infections have decreased; while the immunization rates among children and pregnant woman have increased, with deliveries conducted hygienically, even in remote villages.

Local traditional birth attendants (e.g. *dais,* etc.) are often included early on, and their involvement after some basic training is very important. Similarly, traditional healers can sometimes be involved in primary health care, especially related to maternal and child health.

Money and materials

The well-off and important people in the community, and local and district-level administrative bodies, support part or all the salaries of the primary health workers, provide supplementary foods if required (p.235), buy some of the medicines and build clinic buildings etc. Financial support by the community makes them directly involved and makes for a better performance of the health worker, who is aware of the fact that everyone in the village indirectly contributes towards her or his salary, and that she or he is working for the people, who, in turn, can watch and judge her or his work. The community's organized involvement can also assist in establishing cottage industries, which eventually may help in raising the mother's income, with the increased possibility of buying additional nutritious foods (p.61).

Involvement in maternal and child health care

The community provides a site for the MCH clinic in the form of a building constructed by the people themselves, or part of someone's house, used without charging any rent. They help in collecting children and women for physical check-ups, weighing, immunizations and group feeding of poorly nourished young children and mothers (if indicated). They maintain growth charts of children and help health workers in identifying and looking after children and pregnant women who are 'at risk' because of poverty, large families, previous malnutrition, etc. To those who are poor, the community may be able to provide transportation for referral to the health centre or to the hospital centre.

Involvement in nutrition programmes

Mother-to-mother advice and discussion can help in ensuring the onset and success of breast-feeding, particularly for young mothers in urban areas. Women's organizations or youth clubs can help primary health care workers in watching over the nutrition of children and women by monthly weighing or by measuring the child's arm circumference.

In some places, community participation has developed simple village equipment to prepare 'multimix' nutritious supplementary foods for sale or distribution to mothers and young children. They have promoted community, school and home gardens—all concerned with growing locally important, nutritious foods (p.61). In some programmes, community kitchens have been established where malnourished children and pregnant and lactating mothers receive supplementary feeding daily.

Involvement in child spacing programme

The primary health care worker and the people themselves assist in child-spacing programmes by spreading information and explaining advantages to uncertain couples. In some areas, contraceptives may be made available, as well as advice on referral for infertile couples. The family planning programmes are more successful when community support is obtained.

Disease control

Members of the community can help in organizing immunization programmes, the regular distribution of antimalarial tablets (if indicated), and the distribution and use of oral rehydration packets (p.106), to parents of young children with diarrhoea (p.102). Primary health care workers from the community can provide basic simple treatment for common day-to-day illnesses.

Environmental sanitation

Local people have been involved in building community wells, preparing rooftop rainwater collection tanks and using bamboo pipes in the distribution of water. Youths or schoolchildren can assist in chlorinating drinking water wells or tanks, in some circumstances. One of the clearest examples of community involvement is that of construction of pit latrines and group programmes for the cleaning of the village. In some countries, compost has been used not only as a soil fertilizer, but also for the production of 'biogas' for heating and lighting. In China, community action has succeeded in controlling rats, flies, and some other pests. All these activities lead to improved maternal and child health as well, of course, to the improved health of the community.

Health education by people to the people

Schoolchildren, youths and leaders in the women's organizations can educate and inform others on various aspects of health, immunization and nutrition. The message from a person from the community can assist greatly in changing awareness of problems, attitudes, practices and behaviour (p.190).

Involvement in other activities

In some programmes, the community has organized day care centres for small children where combined activities concerned with health, nutrition and pre-school education have been carried out. At the same time, mothers can be given adult education, including literacy classes, and receive training in village 'cottage industry,' which can give them some income.

Organization of child-to-child programmes

In some places, school-age children have been trained to look after their younger brothers and sisters when their parents go out to work, including teaching about avoiding accidents (p.187), watching out for malnutrition—even using arm-bands to recognize thin limbs—etc.

Supervision

The community has to be involved in the supervision of

primary health care workers, which makes for greater interest in the planning, carrying out and modifying of programmes.

Evaluation

The people should be involved in the collection of information, including measuring health and nutrition using simple means (p.227). This action on the part of the community makes for further understanding and involvement. In particular, they develop a better recognition of their 'real needs' as well as of their previously recognized 'felt needs'.

Further scope

The involvement of the community will vary from area to area according to the local needs, resources, programmes, and the ability of workers in the local health service and other village-improvement agencies to arouse interest. There is often a possibility of quite a wide range of activities, as indicated by the following practical examples.

1. The community can organize the collection of one handful of rice and legumes, or excess of milk or buttermilk, daily for nutrition supplementation programmes. At the time of harvest, those who can afford it should be approached for a small contribution of grain.

2. Indirect ways of promoting nutrition of growing children include methods to increase food production, such as the construction of rat-proof village grain stores, the development of co-operatives and bank loans, Food-For-Work schemes, and other similar activities which should be encouraged through the community's active participation.

3. Health insurance schemes, building 'midwifery huts' and a wide variety of other measures can succeed with community action.

Problems

The health professionals who try to involve communities

should train themselves (and their fellow workers) in the culture of the society (p.12), so that they themselves can fit in with and understand the ways of the local community. They should observe people, talk with them, work with them and appreciate their work. However, such health workers should avoid local 'politics' and should be understanding concerning topics such as religion, customs, beliefs and taboos. It is easier to modify the behaviour of people related to beliefs and customs (p.12), when and if indicated, after gaining their confidence and when they recognize benefits to themselves (p.191).

Friendly co-operation between different governmental officials (agriculture, education, etc.), non-governmental agents (concerned with the welfare of mothers and children), and health workers is also important. Rivalries and not working together can make community action very difficult—or impossible. It is important for the different agencies concerned with village-level improvement—all of which relates to the health of mothers and their children–to have meetings to discuss their activities and ensure that they support each other.

Since the World Health Organization Alma Ata Declaration of 1978, the countries of the world, especially developing countries, have realized that primary health care is the only possible way to reach their populations. Community involvement is an essential part of this different way of looking at improving health, and mothers and young children are priorities.

26
Training

Ashfaq Ahmad

In the tropical developing countries today, most childhood deaths are due to a multitude of infections and malnutrition, each adversely interacting with the other. Most of these could be prevented by the provision of simple curative services close to people's homes, together with preventive measures such as immunization, health supervision, better nutrition, improved sanitation, health education, family planning and raised living standards. Better nutrition and raised living standards are mainly to be solved at the socio-political level. The other measures require widespread use of relatively simple and inexpensive technology.

Special individual medical attention mainly for the urban elite must give place to 'basic health care for all'. A minimal amount of health care is a basic human right, and the modern health team made up of doctors, various types of nurses, and assisted by many auxiliaries must be recognized and used.

A training strategy must be planned related to national health problems and the over-all policy (p.260) concerned with training of all levels of health staff. In planning this strategy, demand for and supply and use of trained staff should be taken into consideration.

Future doctors*

Since the quantity and nature of paediatric problems vary from country to country, and even from year to year, uniform teaching for all areas is neither practicable nor desirable. There is a need for a continuous review of education in child health, with the stress on appropriateness to local problems, on flexibility and on the introduction of new ideas. Child health should be treated as a major subject in the medical curriculum at the undergraduate level. Its study

251

should start from the third year and continue through all the 3 years of clinical training (if this is the local length).

Four hundred hours for undergraduate child health training, with 3 months of compulsory internship, has been recommended in some countries. Out of the proposed 400 hours, 100 hours should be devoted to lectures, the remaining 300 hours to clinical demonstrations, clerkship and other practical work.

Training in child health should not only be confined to hospitals, but must also extend into the home and community. The ecological approach should be emphasized — that is, the role of cultural (p. 12) and environmental factors, such as poverty, an inadequate water supply, village hygiene etc., in the causation of disease should be given due importance.

There should be sufficient emphasis on perinatal medicine (concerning the overlapping problems of the fetus and newborn), and on maternal and child health services. In addition, training must include the usual subjects covered everywhere, but with a much greater emphasis on locally important conditions, especially nutrition, parasitic infections, infectious diseases, etc. Similar considerations apply to training for nurses, midwives and nutritionists.

Auxiliaries

As Dr Mahler (Director of WHO) has said: 'We must be

---

* Due to shortage of trained paediatricians, the successful introduction of the *paediatric nurse practitioner* for providing medical services for children in the understaffed and overcrowded hospitals of the region has occurred in Pakistan. These practitioners are able to screen, diagnose, and provide initial treatment of sick children attending outpatient departments of hospitals. By history taking, physical examination and performance of practical procedures, they should diagnose common paediatric illnesses and apply standard treatments. Similarly, by recognizing those children whose illnesses fall outside their level of knowledge, they can refer them to specialist care after providing emergency treatment. They will also provide preventive and educational services with particular regard to nutrition, immunization, family planning and child health. The paediatric nurse practitioner trainees (male and female) can be chosen after 3 years of nursing practice and should be given 6–9 months intensive training in the above skills.

willing to admit that skills are not given by God only to the physicians or the public health nurse; skills can be taught to virtually anyone to meet local conditions and needs.' The role of auxiliaries in health services for children cannot be over-emphasized; they should be the main force in health service activities to improve child health. They should be trained for the task they are expected to perform, and should receive supervision, support and continuing inservice training.

Central Auxiliary Institute

In some countries, a Central Health Auxiliary Institute (or equivalent) can be established. This can provide training, research and evaluation relating to primary health care services. It can be the site for meeting of a Health Auxiliary Council and other experts who would work out the details of curricula, teaching training, developing a reference library and audio-visual aids, etc.

Training schools

Some of these schools should be placed near teaching hospitals to facilitate in-service training. The number and type of individuals enrolled for different categories should be determined by consideration of the ratio of urban to rural population, the number of hospital beds available for in-patients and the access of a physician (preferably a paediatrician) to supervise treatment and to see referrals. Training of many different types of worker can be carried out together. This has not only economic advantages, but also can foster team spirit and prepare the students for their future working circumstances. Such training schools should also have the responsibility for continuing education and training courses after qualification. Details will vary with circumstances in different countries.

Training methods

Certain subjects which form the basis of common teaching for all the categories, such as the structure and function of the body, nutrition, personal and environmental hygiene and health education etc., should be included in the initial period of teaching. Subjects meant for a particular training programme should be included *according to the work the auxiliary will be doing.*

Systems vary greatly from one country to another, but several categories of auxiliary will be needed, particularly more trained workers, part of whose duties will be supervision and looking after referrals, and village-level primary health care workers.

Supervisory workers

In different countries, there are different supervisory workers with various duties, including public health nurses. In Pakistan, the Lady Health Visitor or the Auxiliary Nurse Midwife has this role.

They (and similar workers in other countries) form the most important link between the doctor and the community and play a main role in the health service. They provide health care and supervision to a considerable population (often about 3000 but varying with local geography), which includes home visiting, often every 3 months.

In Pakistan the training of Lady Health Visitors lasts about 2 years and the entrance requirement is a minimum qualification of 10 years schooling, preferably with science subjects. During this period they should be trained to organize maternity clinics, perform antenatal and postnatal examinations and manage minor obstetrical complications and emergencies.

They should also be taught to run young child clinics (p.224), diagnose and treat common childhood diseases, and refer the unmanageable cases to the paediatrician. They should be able to carry out immunization (p.201) and to undertake nutrition education (p.190).

Apart from receiving training along medical lines, the Lady Health Visitor should be given an understanding of administration and personnel management, of cultural aspects of health (p.12) and methods of communication (p.190).

This would prepare her for working independently in the community and ensure the supervision of the health aides (see below).

Village-level workers

In primary health care services, trained village-level primary health care workers (PHCWs) are needed.

The activities that can be undertaken by PHCWs will plainly vary with local needs and the presence of other extension agents in the community (e.g. from agriculture etc.). A common pattern is that of two PHCWs—one female and one male—in a community, with tasks often related to traditional roles. It seems clear that women will play a major part, not only because of the emphasis on the health care and feeding of mothers and young children, but also because some duties may only be carried out by women in some cultures, and because of the increasing awareness of the role of women in national development.

In all cases, PHCWs need to be part of an existing health system, with opportunities for referral, for supervision, for continuing education and, in some countries, the opportunity for carefully selected experienced workers to receive further training and promotion.

While there can be no universal model and much depends on the PHCW's ability to enlist the participation of the community, the following summary gives a general range of activities which can be undertaken by PHCWs, with suggested minimal activities indicated with an asterisk (*).

1. *Improved food consumption*

Information collection (*). The personal contact, especially during home visits, can insure simple day-to-day observations of usual practices.

Observing the nutrition of mothers and young children (*). Collection by PHCWs of information on *growth* (mainly growth charts, p.227) and of *selected clinical signs and symptoms*, e.g. Bitot's spots (p.97) anaemia (p.83), night blindness (p.97), particularly from those young children and mothers in families known to be at risk.

Health education (*). This is best seen as a two-way exchange of information and advice. It should contain motivation (p.190), be rooted in the indigenous culture (p.12), and involve the use of locally available materials such as foods (or acceptable alternatives). Practical demonstrations are very important, for example with real foods and actual kitchen conditions. The *topics* to be covered would vary with need, but in the nutritional field, would usually include the advantages of breast-feeding (including anti-infective and child-spacing effects etc); home-prepared weaning foods; maternal diet in pregnancy and lactation; correct use of food supplements (when relevant); how to select most economical and nutritious purchased foods (when relevant); how to prevent the main locally important infections; and how to use local services.

Nutritional supplements. If programmes to distribute nutritional supplements are to be included, they need to be *very* carefully defined with regard to real need, and to target groups, indications for issue, cultural acceptability, local availability of foods. Major concerns should be their nutrition education message and encouragement of local food production and use.

Two categories of nutritional supplements may be considered:

(i) *preventive*: oral vitamin A or iron (when indicated),

(ii) *remedial*: usually a food or foods (as a source of calories, protein and other nutrients) for issue for limited periods of time for *young children with flattening weight curves, or for pregnant lactating women with weight loss or inadequate lactation.*

Treatment (*). Basic treatment for the main problems, including malnutrition, should be available. However, severe protein–energy malnutrition, with complications, may often need referral for treatment in hospitals (if such exist), although the risks are nowadays appreciated, especially cross-infection in crowded children's wards and inadequate numbers of staff to care for in-patients. Children with malnutrition can often be treated in nutrition rehabilitation units (or similar, less formally organized feeding centres), or in their own homes.

Child spacing. The health and nutrition of young children and the amount of food available to families are reduced by child spacing. Activities by the PHCW can vary greatly in different cultural circumstances from *arousing awareness* (*), to *motivating and referring*, to actual *distribution of acceptable contraceptives.*

2. *Improved food utilization*

'Food utilization' is here used in a special sense—to include the body's ability to absorb nutrients and to avoid losing them as a result of infections.

Increased food absorption. The PHCW can assist by emphasizing improved traditional methods of milling, grinding, sieving and cooking which make weaning foods easier and/or cheaper to prepare and more digestible (*), and hence absorbed into the body.

Infections: General. Gastrointestinal, insect-borne and other infections or nutritional consequence can be reduced by the PHCW trying to assist in developing an *adequate water supply* and *simple, but effective, waste disposal*, and by village-level approaches to *decreasing insect breeding.*

Infections: specific. Prevention. This will always include *health education* (*) (geared to personal and home hygiene, and major infections), together with referral for *appropriate immunization* (*) (especially whooping cough, measles, tuberculosis) and, in affected areas, the distribution of *antimalarials* (*) (for pregnant women and children during the 'weaning period').

Treatment. Varying levels of treatment may be advisable, feasible and permissible, particularly medicines for everyday minor illnesses (e.g. colds, aches and pains, cuts etc.), '*deworming*'(*) (with piperazine), and *oral rehydration*(*).

3. *Improved food supplies*

The PHCW must be *aware* of the great importance of sufficent supplies of the main foods in the community, of the need for joining with other extension agents (e.g. from agriculture etc.), and of the need to *collect information*(*) on the local food situation by simple observation, both for foods grown and those imported into village shops.

4. *Improved income*

When possible, the PHCW can *encourage and assist* in *special activities producing income*, especially for women, and should *encourage efforts towards economically helpful community activities* (e.g. village-level food processing).

A major concern is always to try to avoid the PHCW becoming overloaded with an impossible number of tasks. Selection is the key, depending on the community's own felt needs and knowledge of the most serious family health and nutrition problems in the area, and the ease of prevention.

> *Pakistan example.* In Pakistan, PHWCs are called 'health aides', They work at the village level as health motivators, obtainers of health information (e.g. concerning epidemics) and informants concerning village resources for health services, as well as providing health education. Health aides also provide nutrition surveillance of young children by regular weighing, and manage a selected list of common health problems by the use of a small drug supply. In certain countries of the region like Pakistan and India, one type of health aide is a trained indigenous midwife, who is a female. The scope of her work can be enlarged, so that she becomes competent in the above-mentioned skills in addition to conducting deliveries for which she already been trained.
>
> In many developing countries, there is a pool of drop-outs from schools after primary education, especially between the eighth and tenth years of education. In Pakistan and elsewhere, these individuals can be enrolled into training schools and, after a period of 1 year during which they are taught the basics, they may be attached to a maternity and child health centre for a further period of 8 months. After this period, they are qualified health aides and can work in the community.

Community health workers, including religious leaders, social workers, school teachers etc., can be given basic training in improving the health of mothers and their children. These individuals working on a voluntary basis can assist the health aides and, through their close understanding of the community, they can undertake health education and motivate the public to adopt practices to improve family health.

Conclusion

Health care services require sufficient manpower (or really human power, as women will probably be mostly needed), which must suit the needs of a community. The examples given here are often based on experience in Pakistan. Similar principles can be used elsewhere, but with different categories and roles to suit different circumstances. The aim is to provide trainees with appropriate practical technical skills and competence to work in their particular settings.

Training should be practical and, for PHCWs, as near to the home area as possible. Examinations also should be concerned with the trainees' ability to work in real-life conditions rather than being a test of their ability to memorize. When appropriate, opportunities may be available for health workers to advance from one level to another after considerable experience and further training.

The child population in the tropics is large and medical services limited. The purpose of appropriate training for all levels of workers is to organize a network of child care service, in the hospital, the health centre and the village, taking into consideration limited funds, cultural differences, and the geographical situation.

27
Child health policy

Mamdouh M. Gabr

A workable child health policy—that is, an agreed upon national plan—has to be considered as part of each country's development policy, designed to improve the social and economic situation for the nation. A child health policy also has to be part of a government's general health policy.

A child health policy does not have the same priority in every country. Moreover, some activities which do not on the surface seem to be 'child health policies' should indeed be included. For example, a most important aspect of child health policy in many developing countries is concerned with population and family planning. Policies to decrease rapid population growth also attempt to ensure that children will have a better chance for living and growing normally. Child health policy should be part of a general policy *between* ministries: a complete child health policy cannot, for example, ignore the great importance of environmental sanitation, income levels, availability of food, socio-cultural practices, beliefs and taboos. Some of these may be more affected by policies of various ministries, including the Ministry of Health.

Once a policy and its aims have been decided on, a plan of action has to be agreed to, carefully selecting from the different approaches ('strategies') available.

Plan of action

In considering a plan of action, the following need attention.

1. 'Technical feasibility' (availability of practical scientific methods suitable for the local situation).

2. 'Appropriate technology' (availability of economical, simple apparatus, etc.).

3. 'Political, community and cultural acceptability'.

4. 'Absorptive capacity' (possibility of carrying out the plan with locally producible staff, equipment, etc.).

5. 'Cost-effectiveness' (value of activities compared with their benefit, bearing in mind other methods).

The 'at-risk' approach is a good starting point in considering priorities. For example, in countries with very low infant mortalities, high incomes and industrialization, problems of the handicapped and the emotionally disturbed children may be in the 'high-risk' group and need a relatively high priority. However, in settings where infant mortalities are high and where children who do live are faced with very many serious problems just to keep alive and without disease, rehabilitation services cannot be given a high priority.

Policy and choices in developing countries should be based on their problems and what they need, not on what other countries do.

After agreeing to strategies and a plan of action, the methods and services through which programmes will be delivered need to be considered, as do ways of checking their effectiveness (evaluation).

Evaluation requires establishment of criteria (or agreed facts) on which to judge effectiveness—these can indicate how well services are delivered (e.g. number of children reached), *or* how much health has improved, *or*, preferably, both. Information on deaths and illness is an important indicator of the health of a community. Evaluation of health services including their availability, nearness and acceptability to the population, is obviously important.

Child health and national development

Health is a vital part of any national development policy aimed at improving the quality of life of all citizens. Infant and childhood illness and deaths represent the main health problem in developing countries. Social and economic development can help in lowering the mortality in such countries.

Also, the healthy development of children is important to national development.

Principles of child health policy

Improvement in health cannot be gained by action by the Ministry of Health alone. Contributions from other sectors, such as agriculture, food production, education, housing and water supply, all have important effects on the health of the population. The widespread use of simple, preferably locally made, technology—such as growth charts (p.227), cheap weighing scales (p.230), arm circumference tapes—can have a much greater effect on maternal and child health than sophisticated and expensive technology limited to medical centres in cities. Each country should define an overall health policy, and within this policy give the highest priority to the strengthening of maternal and child health services in the following ways.

1. Attention should be given to providing services to deal with the main health needs of mothers and children, based on a carefully thought-out strategy and plan of action.

2. Discussion should be held with staff at all levels of the health service to ensure that the policy is understood and carried out, once it has been developed and approved.

3. In developing a child health policy, all appropriate sectors (mainly ministries) should be involved, particularly health, education, agriculture and community development. A means for discussion, exchange of views and working together (co-ordination) needs to be established in any country.

Evaluation

A method for evaluation of child health services should be set up. The following factors should be considered.

1. *Coverage*: percentage of the population in different areas reached by primary health care workers and others,

supervised deliveries, attendance, postnatal clinics, family planning advice, immunization and numbers reached by infant and preschool child services.

2. *Nutrition* of children under 2 years of age and occurrence of *anaemia* in pregnancy.

3. *Mortality*, especially infant and young child (1–4 years) mortalities.

The development of a system to provide appropriate and *timely* information is essential, both for planning and evaluation. Eventually, the system in each country should be improved to obtain more sensitive indicators of child health, including, for example, prematurity and stillbirth rates.

Manpower development and training
(see also p.251)

The more readily identifiable problems related to trained manpower to run the health services often include the following.

1. The uneven distribution of specialized and other professional services between urban and rural areas.

2. The scarcity of certain types of personnel, e.g. public health nurses, nutrition specialists and health educators.

3. The inadequacy and inappropriateness of training programmes for the local situation.

4. Failure to define clearly the duties of different types of health worker.

5. Lack of real awareness of the need for, and practical training of, *large numbers* of primary health care workers.

Guidelines describing the duties of individual types of health workers should be prepared and brought into action. Traditional birth attendants (TBAs), can be identified and trained and can then undertake other duties, such as referrals, follow-ups and notifications of births and deaths. Villagers who can work as community health aides can be identified and trained to carry out duties as needed. Efforts should be made to improve both the quantity and quality of training, with special emphasis on primary health care workers.

Community participation

Community participation is essential to the health of people
(p.244). Emphasis in health education (p.187) should be given
to the advantages of breast-feeding (p.56), to beneficial
weaning practices (p.15), the use of locally produced
nutritious foods (often as multimixes, p.61), the improved
preparation and storage of locally grown foods, the
prevention of infections (p.   ), etc. Governments should
make greater use of mass media to promote improved health
practices (p.197), including the wise use of purchased foods
(consumer education).

Maternal health care

Child health services cannot be considered without also giving
attention to maternal health services (p.215). These should
include the care of the pregnant woman, the safe delivery of
her child, her postnatal supervision, the care of the newborn
infant, the maintenance of breast-feeding, and family
planning. The level of maternal health in a community is
generally estimated by information on ill-health and deaths in
pregnancy and childbirth, on the commonness of low-birth-
weight babies and still-births, and on deaths of babies just
after birth.

'High-risk' pregnancies (e.g. poor weight gain, anaemia,
etc.) should be identified by the health staff (p.215), and
these mothers should receive the additional care needed for
their particular condition. The health and nutrition of the
pregnant mothers should be specially looked at (p.215) and
corrected, when necessary. Health education (p.188) to
pregnant mothers is an important part of antenatal care.
When possible and needed, immunization of pregnant
mothers against tetanus should be carried out for the
prevention of tetanus neonatorum in their babies (p.211).

The main concern during childbirth is to ensure that every

woman has a safe delivery with the least possible risk to herself and to her baby. As many deliveries as possible should be attended by trained health workers, including trained traditional birth attendants (TBAs). All women with a likelihood of a difficult delivery should be admitted to a maternity unit with appropriate staff and equipment.

Normal deliveries can be conducted at home by the well-trained midwife, provided there is adequate space and reasonable surroundings and light. The nurse or midwife attending the delivery should be provided with suitable equipment and should have access to emergency services for referral in case complications take place during delivery. Reasons for referral should be clearly understood.

Every effort should be made to encourage breast-feeding as soon as possible after birth. The weight of the newborn baby should be taken. Special arrangements should be made available to transport very low-birth-weight babies born at home to a hospital, when such exists.

Postnatal care is very important for both mother and child. Meetings with the mother can provide a good opportunity for discussion and education concerning her own health and the infant's needs, as well as child spacing (p.217). When practicable, home visits should be carried out during the first 10 days. A postnatal examination is advisable, not later than 6 weeks after delivery, when discussion and arranging for family planning may be well received by the mother.

Preschool child health care

Services for young children aim at ensuring the healthy development of the 0–5-year-old child, including checking growth and development using weight charts (p.227), and, in some cases, checking 'milestones' for motor and psychological development (p.25). All children should receive immunization against preventable diseases—diptheria, whooping cough, tetanus, measles, polio and tuberculosis (p.135). Promotion of breast-feeding is essential in preventing malnutrition (p.65) and diarrhoea (p.102) in young infants. The use of locally produced nutritionally and culturally acceptable foods during the weaning period is essential (p.61). Diarrhoea is a major cause of death in children thoughout the developing world, and is also a major cause in producing malnutrition. Deaths due to diarrhoeal diseases could be reduced greatly through the immediate use of oral rehydration (p.106), which can be carried out within the family, thus greatly increasing its widespread use. Early identification and treatment of minor diseases in the family and community significantly reduce mortality and serious illness. Coverage should be increased by all possible means, and out-reach services planned and carried out, especially using primary health care services (p.215). 'High-risk' children have to be identified and given the appropriate care or increased observation. 'At-risk' indicators should be identified for each community, so that these families or individual children can be supervised especially carefully.

Health of schoolchildren (see also p.238)

Attendance at school constitutes the first opportunity to screen somewhat older children for important health problems and to make good any inadequate health supervision in the preschool group.

Ideally, a school health programme should include the following (but has to be limited by the availability of funds, staff and services to which children can be referred): the detection of health defects, the improvement of the school environment, a school meal service, a booster immunisation programme and child and parent guidance services as well as family-life education, including information on family planning, nutrition, sex education and breast-feeding. However, limited funds usually make this a rather neglected group, and certainly priority problems occur in infancy and the preschool age. Further discussion of school health services is given elsewhere (p.238).

Appendix: Paediatric Drug Dosage

This is a list of drugs used commonly in the treatment of young children. Local variation in dosage may be necessary and the strength of available tablets and mixtures must be known. Treatment should always be as simple as possible, and great care must be taken to make sure that mothers really understand when and how to give drugs on return home.

Adrenaline	1 : 1000 solution in water 0.01 ml/kg per dose to maximum 0.5 ml subcutaneously
Aminophylline	4 mg/kg per dose i.v. (slowly); 6 mg/kg per dose rectally. May be repeated 4-hourly
Ampicillin	50 mg/kg per 24 hours given 6-hourly Higher doses up to 400 mg/kg in meningitis
Aspirin	Soluble tablets: 300 mg 12.5 mg/kg as a single dose Not more than 50 mg/kg per 24 hours (higher dose for rheumatic fever) Under 5 years of age, suggest paracetamol
Chloral hydrate	Mild sedation: 30 mg/kg per dose Heavy sedation: 60 mg/kg per dose
Chloramphenicol	Capsules: 250 mg 50 mg/kg per 24 hours given 6-hourly Higher doses up to 200 mg/kg in severe infections, but reduce after 48 hours In the newborn, reduce to 25 mg/kg per 24 hours for first month

i.v. = intravenously; i.m. = intramuscularly; i.t. = intrathecally.

267

Chlorpromazine
(Largactil)   1 mg/kg per dose orally, i.m. or i.v.
                       In neonatal tetanus, 2–4 mg/kg per dose

Chloroquine   Subcutaneously (rarely i.m.) 5 mg/kg per
                       dose
                       By mouth 1 tablet = 100 mg
                       Years   Tablets per day for 3 days
                       0–1   ¼
                       1–5   ½
                       6–10   **1**
                       Over 10   **2**
                       **Prophylaxis: weekly doses on the same
                       scale**

Cloxacillin   50 mg/kg per 24 hours given 6-hourly

Codeine phosphate   Linctus BPC (adult) contains 15 mg
                       codeine phosphate/5 ml
                       Linctus paediatric contains 3 mg codeine
                       phosphate/5 ml
                       Single dose 0.25 mg/kg
                       Not more than four doses/24 hours
                       Do not give to children under 1 year of
                       age

Co-trimoxazole (Septrin
Bactrim)   1 part trimethoprim and 5 parts
                       sulphamethoxazole
                       Dose expressed as sum of trimethoprim
                       and sulphamethoxazole (new convention)
                       Tablet (paediatric): 120 mg
                       Suspension (paediatric): 240 mg/5 ml
                       i.v. ampoules: 480 mg/5 ml, must be
                       diluted
                       48 mg/kg per 24 hours by mouth in two
                       doses

Diazepam (Valium)   In convulsions: 0.25 mg/kg per dose i.v.,
                       repeated 1–3-hourly as necessary

Maintenance: 0.2 mg/kg per 24 hours
given 6-hourly i.v. or by intragastric tube
Higher doses are often needed in neonatal
tetanus

Dichlorophen (An-   4–6 g, single dose
tiphen)

Digoxin   Elixir: 0.05 mg/ml
Tablets: 0.0625 mg, 0.125 mg and 0.25 mg
Injection ampoules: 0.1 mg in 1 ml and
0.5 mg in 2 ml
Total digitalizing dose: 0.04 mg/kg per 24
hours in three or four doses
For rapid digitalization: half total 24-hour
dose stat i.m., quarter total 24-hour dose
in 6 and 12 hours
Maintenance: 0.01 mg/kg per 24 hours
N.B. Watch carefully the position of the
decimal point. A ten times error in the
dose may be lethal.

Emetine hydrochloride   1 mg/kg per 24 hours
Give 12-hourly deep subcutaneously

Ephedrine   2.5 mg/kg per 24 hours in three doses

Erythromycin   50 mg/kg per 24 hours given 6-hourly by
mouth or i.v.
Dose may be doubled

Ferrous sulphate   Tablets: 200 mg contains 60 mg iron
Mixture: 60 mg (18 mg iron) in 5 ml
20 mg/kg per 24 hours in three doses by
mouth

Flucloxacillin   50 mg/kg per 24 hours
Give 6-hourly i.v. or by mouth
Twice as easily absorbed as cloxacillin

Folic acid   Tablets: 5 mg
0.25 mg/kg per 24 hours

Frusemide (Lasix)   1 mg/kg per 24 hours in single dose
May be repeated once

Furozolidone (Furox-   6 mg/kg per 24 hours given 6-hourly by
one)   mouth

Gentamicin   i.v./i.m. ampoules: 20 mg and 80 mg/2
ml
Intrathecal (i.t.): 5 mg/ml
i.m./i.v. 6 mg/kg per 24 hours in three
doses
i.t.: 2 mg/24 hours in a single dose

Hydrocortisone   Ampoules: 100 mg, 500 mg i.m., i.v.
50–100 mg as a single dose
Repeatable 6-hourly

Iron dextran (Imferon)   50 mg iron/ml
Injections should be deep i.m.
Total requirement = (lack of Hb as a
percentage $\times$ body weight in kg $\times$ 0.15)
mg iron.
Can be given i.v. but see manufacturer's
instruction.

Isoniazid (INH, INAH)   Prophylaxis in neonates: 5 mg/kg per 24
hours
10–20 mg/kg per day in a single dose
(maximum 300 mg)

Mebendazole   Tablets: 100 mg (can be chewed)
Suspension: 100 mg/5 ml
100 mg daily for 3 days
Do not give to children under 2 years of
age

Mepacrine   Tablets: 100 mg
     Giardiasis   0–2 years: 25
mg/dose
2–5 years: 50
mg/dose
Two doses daily for 5 days

| | *Tapeworms* | 2–5 years: 400 mg
6–10 years: 600 mg
Over 10 years: 800 mg |

Metronidazole (Flagyl)   Tablets: 200 mg (also suppositories: 500 mg)
Suspension: 200 mg in 5 ml
Injection: 5 mg/ml in 100-ml bottles or 20-ml ampoules
15–50 mg/kg per 24 hours orally in three doses, the larger doses for giardiasis
22.5 mg/kg per 24 hours orally, i.v. infusion for treatment of anaerobic infections
500–1500 mg/24 hours by suppository in three doses from 1–12 years old

Neomycin   50 mg/kg per 24 hours given 6-hourly by mouth

Nitrofurantoin   Tablets: 50 mg
(Furadantin)   Suspension: 25 mg/5 ml
                           6 mg/kg per 24 hours given 6 hourly

Nystatin (Mycostatin)   Tablets: 500 000 units
                           Suspension: 100 000 units/ml
                           Newborn and infants: 400 000 units/24 hours given 6-hourly
                           Older children: 1–2 million units/24 hours

Paracetamol (Calpol)   Tablets: 500 mg
                           Elixir: 120 mg/5 ml
                           15 mg/kg per dose
                           Not more than four doses in 24 hours

Paraldehyde   (1 g/ml) 0.15–0.3 ml/kg per dose i.m.
                           By rectum, 0.6 ml/kg per dose

Para-aminosalicylic   250 mg/kg per day, divided into three
(PAS)   doses

Penicillin
Type   *Soluble* i.m., i.v.   *Procaine* i.m.
                           1 mega unit = 600   300 000 units (300
                           mg   mg)/ml

Frequency of dose	i.m. 4–12-hourly i.v. infusion	once daily
Dose: under 7 years	300 mg (0.5 mega units)/kg per 24 hours	0.5 ml/kg per 24 hours
Dose: over 7 years	600 mg (1 mega unit)/kg per 24 hours	1.0 ml/kg per 24 hours
Dose: neonates	30 mg/kg per 24 hours	0.05 ml/kg per 24 hours

Very much higher doses in meningitis

Type	*Triplopen* i.m.	*V. oral*
Frequency of dose	every 3 days 2 mega units/vial	4–6 hourly 125 mg/5 ml 125–250 mg/tablets
Dose: under 7 years	¼ vial	62.5–125 mg
Dose: over 7 years	½ vial	250 mg

Pethidine
Tablets: 25 mg, 50 mg
i.v. injection: 50 mg/ml
1 mg/kg by mouth or i.m., single dose
Dose may be doubled in severe pain

Phenobarbitone
Tablets: 7.5 mg, 15 mg, 30 mg and 60 mg
Elixir: 15 mg in 5 ml
Injection: 30 mg, 60 mg and 200 mg/ml
Sedation: 3 mg/kg per dose
Anticonvulsant: 6 mg/kg per dose i.m.
Maintenance: 6 mg/kg per 24 hours
Given 12-hourly by mouth

Phenytoin (Epanutin)
Tablets: 50 mg
Capsules: 50 mg and 100 mg
Mixture: 30 mg/5 ml
i.v. ampoule: 250 mg/5 ml (5 mg/ml)
6 mg/kg per 24 hours in two doses
5–10 mg/kg i.v. in single dose, 1 mg/kg per minute

Piperazine
Under 2 years: 2 g
2–5 years: 3 g

Over 5 years: 4 g
Single dose repeated in 2 days if no
worms passed

Prednisolone   Tablets: 1 mg, 5 mg, 25 mg
                          2 mg/kg per 24 hours three times daily
                          In asthma: reduce dose after severe attack
                          relieved, and discontinue as soon as
                          possible (within 10 days)

Promethazine   Tablets: 10 mg, 25 mg
(Phenergan)   Syrup: 5 mg/5 ml
                          1 mg/kg per dose up to three times daily

Rifampicin   Capsules: 150 mg, 300 mg
                          Suspension: 100 mg/5 ml
                          15 mg/kg once daily
                          Only for use in tuberculosis

Salbutamol (Ventolin)   Tablets: 2 mg, 4 mg
                          Syrup: 2 mg/5 ml
                          Nebulizer solution: 5 mg/ml; dilute in
                          normal saline or water
                          Injection: 500 mcg/ml (1000 mcg = 1 mg)
                          Infusion i.v.: 5 mg/5 ml
                          0.4 mg/kg per 24 hours by mouth in three
                          or four doses
                          2–5 mg/24 hours by nebulizer
                          4 mcg/kg per 24 hours i.v. as a single dose
                          0.6 mcg/kg per hour i.v. as continuous
                          infusion

Streptomycin   Infants: 20 mg/kg;
                          others: 40 mg/kg per 24 hours i.m.
                          Divide 12-hourly
                          In TB, give single dose daily
                          Intrathecal dose 1 mg/kg per 24 hours

Sulphadimidine   Tablets: 0.5 g
                          100-200 mg/kg per 24 hours given
                          6-hourly
                          Not used in newborns

Tetrachlorethylene	0.1 ml/kg per dose Maximum 5 ml, given in one dose
Tetracycline	Capsules: 250 mg 25 mg/kg per 24 hours given 6-hourly Not used in newborns
Thiacetazone (Tbl)	Combined with isoniazid as 50 mg thiacetazone and 133 mg isoniazid

Under 10 kg	25 mg/day
10–20 kg	50 mg/day
20–40 kg	100 mg/day
Over 40 kg	150 mg/day

Thiamine	50 mg i.m. in single dose, followed by 10 mg daily by mouth in acute beri-beri
Vitamin A	Tablets: 50 000 units (as acetate) Capsules: 4000 units in oil by mouth i.m. injection in water Children at risk of acute deficiency: 100 000–200 000 units daily by mouth for 4 days In keratomalacia: 100 000 units i.m. followed by oral dosage for 4 days

Approximate weights

Where possible, all children should be weighed to ensure accurate dosage. The following are only approximations.

Birth	2.75 kg (6 lb)
4 months	5.5 kg (12 lb)
1 year	8.25 kg (18 lb)
2 years	11 kg (24 lb)
3 years	14 kg (30 lb)

Further reading

BASCH, P. F. (1978). *International Health*. Oxford University Press, New York

BEATON, G. H. and BENGOA, J. M. (eds.) (1976). *Nutrition in Preventive Medicine*. WHO, Geneva.

BRYANT, J. (1969). *Health and the Developing World*. Cornell University Press, Ithaca.

EBRAHIM, G. (1978) *A Handbook of Tropical Paediatrics*. Macmillan, London.

HENDRICKSE, R. (ed) (1981). *Paediatrics in the Tropics: A Current Review*. Oxford University Press, Oxford.

HOVANDER, Y. and CAMERON, M. (1982). *Manual on Feeding of Infants and Young Children*, 3rd edition. United Nations, New York.

JELLIFFE, D. B. and JELLIFFE, E. F. P. (1978). *Human Milk in the Modern World*. Oxford University Press, Oxford.

JELLIFFE, D. B. and JELLIFFE, E. F. P. (1984). *Child Nutrition in Developing Countries*, 2nd edition. USAID, Washington DC.

JELLIFFE, D. B. and JELLIFFE, E. F. P. (1985). *Community Nutrition Assessment*. Oxford University Press, Oxford.

JELLIFFE, D. B. and STANFIELD, J. P. (eds.) (1980). *Diseases of Children in the Subtropics and Tropics*, 3rd edition. Edward Arnold, London.

KING, M., KING, F. and MARTODIPOERO, S. (1978). *Primary Child Care*. Oxford University Press, Oxford.

MORLEY, D. (1973). *Paediatric Priorities in the Tropics*. Butterworth, London.

WILLIAMS, C. D., BAUMSLAG, N. and JELLIFFE, D. B. (1985). *Mother and Child Health: Delivering the Services*. 2nd edition. Oxford University Press, Oxford.

Index